THE NURSE
AND THE
MENTAL PATIENT

A Study in
INTERPERSONAL RELATIONS

By **MORRIS S. SCHWARTZ**, Ph.D.
EMMY LANNING SHOCKLEY, R.N.
M.S. in Nursing Education

With the assistance of
CHARLOTTE GREEN SCHWARTZ, M.A.

NEW YORK • 1956

**RUSSELL SAGE
FOUNDATION**

© 1956
RUSSELL SAGE FOUNDATION
Printed in the United States
of America

Printed May, 1956
Reprinted November, 1956
Reprinted September, 1957

Library of Congress
Catalog Card Number: 56–7932

WM. F. FELL CO., PRINTERS
PHILADELPHIA, PA.

Contents

3

Foreword

TODAY mental hospitals are striving to develop a philosophy of institutional management and of patient care at the ward level that will create a more favorable climate for therapy. This attempt appears to be a renewed emphasis upon ideas prevalent in the earliest days of American psychiatry. More than one hundred years ago Dr. Samuel Woodward, at the Worcester State Hospital, and Dr. John S. Butler, at the Boston State Hospital, developed an atmosphere of warmth and security for their patients and stressed the importance of close personal contact with them.

Within recent years the importance of creating a therapeutic community in the mental hospital has been emphasized by Maxwell Jones in England. Stanton and Schwartz have called attention to the influence of interpersonal relationships in the mental hospital. Caudill, Hyde, Greenblatt, York, and Brown have also reported on their studies made in mental hospitals, which confirm the importance of the hospital atmosphere, attitudes of employees, and relationships between staff and patients in influencing ward behavior and outcome of mental illness.

The need for practical assistance with daily ward problems that arise in every mental institution is everywhere felt. What do nurses and attendants or aides do? They get patients up in the morning, see that they wash, brush their teeth, and go to meals. They make sure patients get enough to eat and that they return to the wards safely. Next, the wards must be cleaned, beds made, and fresh linens obtained from the Central Linen Room. Patients must be bathed, sent for hair-cuts, shaves, or beauty care. Clothing may have to be replaced; a new patient on the ward may require outfitting. The largest task of all is getting patients to scheduled appointments: to the x-ray department or dental clinic, psychological studies, individual or group therapy; also to a treatment room for medicines, electric shock, or insulin, and to occupational therapy or jobs in hospital industries. Then, there is the sick patient with a cold or infection who needs attention. Soon again it is time for meals, and the cycle is repeated. Nursing personnel are always busy.

Things often do not go smoothly; sometimes the day begins with a problem such as a patient's refusing to get out of bed. What does the attendant or nurse do now? Force him to get out of bed or let him miss his breakfast? Suppose on the way to the cafeteria two patients argue as to who is first in line and begin to punch each other. Does the attendant step in between them and risk getting struck himself and his uniform torn, or does he step back and let the patients fight it out until both have black eyes? What does the attendant do if the patient sits on the cafeteria floor with his tray? Does he force the patient to sit at a table? Does he ask the patient politely to move and if he does not, let him sit there? What about the patient who refuses to put his room in order, or will not bathe or shave? Does the attendant struggle with him and hold him down? Or does he use his best efforts at persuasion? What does the nursing staff do about the patient who tears blankets, wets his bed, or sits all day long in a chair with his head bowed, never speaking to anyone? Should very ill mental patients be threatened or punished to exact compliance with rules and appropriate conduct? Should rewards, privileges, and praise be used as incentives?

We know that patients are people, and we sometimes remember that employees are, too. People suffer from insecurity, unmet needs, anxieties, tensions, frustrations, and hostilities, but their degree and manifestations differ from person to person. Ward nursing personnel would like a rule book dealing in precise fashion with problems such as those noted above, and outlining what to do in (1), (2), and (3) fashion. I doubt whether such a rule book would be very helpful even if someone did try to write it, because people are too complex to oblige us by falling into patterned responses.

Success in caring for patients, however, is not merely a matter of chance and of trial-and-error. There is a growing body of concepts and methods that, when published, should do much to answer the constant plea of nursing personnel for help in the development of skills to meet everyday problems. This book by Dr. Morris S. Schwartz and Professor Emmy Lanning Shockley presents simply and realistically a most helpful method for the development of such skills. While the experimental work on which it is based was carried out in a small, well-staffed private mental hospital, the procedure described will prove equally valuable in large, understaffed public institutions.

The basic approach offered is an attempt to understand the meaning of symptoms of mental illness and the significance of behavior through conferences of nursing personnel. Such down-to-earth problems are discussed as: being afraid of a patient, handling the demanding patient, giving recognition to the withdrawn patient, feeding difficulties, dealing with the incontinent, hostile, or seductive patient. If every nurse and aide would read this book and institute the same procedure for trying to understand the needs of those persons entrusted to his or her care, how wonderful it would be for our patients!

WALTER E. BARTON, M.D.

Superintendent, Boston State Hospital,
and Associate Professor of Psychiatry,
Boston University Medical School

Preface

FOR many years nurses have sought to improve their understanding of the emotional as well as the physical needs of the persons under their care. As Dean Elizabeth S. Bixler of the Yale School of Nursing has observed in a recent letter commenting on the manuscript of this book, recognized need for increased understanding has resulted in the case-study approach in schools of nursing, the inclusion of psychiatric nursing in the curriculum, and attempts to integrate concepts from psychiatry and the social sciences into clinical courses. Essential to the continued growth of such understanding are teaching materials—as yet too few—that focus attention in a practical way upon the social-psychological aspects of nursing.

It is with gratification, therefore, that Russell Sage Foundation is publishing *The Nurse and the Mental Patient* by Dr. Morris S. Schwartz and Professor Emmy Lanning Shockley, a sociologist and a psychiatric nurse whose professional experience makes them unusually well equipped for this joint undertaking. The book has been enhanced by a wealth of concrete illustration drawn primarily from a year of research of "what went on" between staff and patients on one of the disturbed wards of a small psychiatric hospital. As the authors indicate, the book has been prepared expressly for those who work with the mentally ill. It is believed that it can be of great helpfulness particularly in discussion groups with nurses and attendants who are undertaking psychiatric nursing for the first time, as well as those who have had considerable experience with patients.

But it is also believed that many of the concepts and attitudes set down are almost equally useful to all nursing. Emphasis, for

9

example, is placed on the fact that the nurse has feelings as well as the patient; that there is continual interaction between the two, the behavior of each influencing the reaction of the other. To quote from Dean Bixler's letter, "In much of our work we are inclined to forget that nurses too are people!" She might have added that nursing education is only at the beginning of helping nurses in any systematic way to handle their feelings and behavior constructively for the benefit of patients and themselves.

Particularly important for nursing as a whole is the method suggested in this book for examining and managing clinical problems. The authors recognize that there may be many ways of dealing with a particular situation, and that there is no one "right" mode of behavior toward all ill patients or even toward the same patient at different times. What they do stress, however, is the fact that there are helpful guides for coping with any situation. These guides include: careful observation by the nurse of her own and the patient's feelings and behavior; appraisal of the therapeutic effects of the procedures being used; exploration of alternate ways of working with him; evaluation of the success of changes made; and further exploration, alterations, and appraisal as indicated.

Finally, the repeated emphasis placed throughout this book on the importance of the therapeutic role of the nurse should furnish much reassurance and support to the nursing profession. To the degree that recognition is accorded such a role, meaning will be given to the status of the nurse as a professional person and a definite goal toward which to work will be provided.

As indicated by the title, this study is concerned exclusively with interpersonal relations as one extremely important aspect of patient care. Nursing procedures and techniques, as traditionally defined, have been omitted since they are the subject of an already extensive literature. Also omitted has been discussion of the effect of the organizational structure of the hospital upon therapeutic undertakings. So potentially important to the success of patient care does organizational structure appear that a brief explanation of its omission from the text is offered.

In recent years sociologists and others who have attempted to study the hospital as a social institution have been increasingly impressed by the degree to which interpersonal relations are facilitated or hindered by the organization of the ward on which the nurse works and of the hospital as a total unit. They have also become interested in the extent to which the physical facilities on the ward and elsewhere in the hospital may be used for therapeutic purposes.

It had been the original intention of the authors to include a discussion of the ways whereby the social context of the hospital influences and shapes relations between patients and personnel. Such discussion would have doubled the size of the book. More important, however, is the fact that materials could not have been presented with any such wealth of illustration as is offered in these pages. Omission of this subject which complements that of interpersonal relations should not leave the impression that its importance in contributing to or limiting the nurse's therapeutic effectiveness has been minimized or underestimated. The social context of psychiatric institutions has received considerable attention of late from several writers, including Dr. Alfred H. Stanton and Dr. Schwartz in *The Mental Hospital*, Basic Books, New York, 1954. In *From Custodial to Therapeutic Patient Care in Mental Hospitals*, published by Russell Sage Foundation in 1955, Dr. Milton Greenblatt, Dr. Richard H. York, and Dr. Esther Lucile Brown have described how experimental modifications in hospital organization permitted appreciable improvement in ward patient care. Still needed, however, is a companion to this book that would present the effect of hospital organization on staff nursing in the immediately useful manner that has been employed here.

ESTHER LUCILE BROWN, PH.D.
Russell Sage Foundation

Introduction

OUR point of view toward nursing the mentally ill was developed in a small mental hospital. The hospital has approximately seventy in-patients, the large majority of whom are diagnosed schizophrenic. One author, a research sociologist and social psychologist, was a participant observer in the hospital, studying and analyzing the relations between doctors, nurses, and patients. In addition, he taught graduate nurses during their field experience at the hospital and supervised various research projects they undertook. The other author, a psychiatric nurse and formerly director of nursing education at the hospital, has been nursing mental patients and teaching student nurses over a period of ten years. She also has planned for and supervised graduate students in their field experience in psychiatric nursing.

This book grew out of a research project carried out on the disturbed ward of the hospital by the sociologist in collaboration with the ward staff during 1952 and 1953. In this project an attempt was made to examine the ways in which nurses relate to patients and to alter these relationships to improve patient mental health. Our examples come primarily from this study and represent real incidents. The sociologist observed directly or participated in and made notes on many of the incidents. Others he learned about in individual and group conferences which were tape-recorded. Still others the nurse-author contributed from her teaching experiences. Because we selected specific case materials for the purpose of illustrating certain points, the examples we present are not necessarily typical of nursing at the hospital. Similarly, the point of view and interpretations are the sole responsibilities of the authors and do not necessarily reflect the hospital's approach to nursing the mentally ill or its interpretation of what might be therapeutic for patients.

The ward we studied housed patients least able to care for themselves in a conventional way and most prone to injure themselves or others. It ordinarily had fifteen patients and was staffed with one head nurse, two to four nurses or aides, and one to three student nurses on the day shift, approximately one regular staff member fewer and one student fewer on the evening shift, and two regular personnel on the night shift. In this situation there was much greater opportunity for nurses and aides to have numerous contacts with patients in a direct, personal, and intensive way than is possible in most mental hospitals. We believe, however, that the processes and problem situations that arose and the interpersonal relations that were carried on by patients and staff were not very different from those in other mental hospitals. This belief is supported by our own experiences in large mental hospitals and reports we have received from others who have worked in many kinds of mental institutions. We further believe that our point of view and approach to problems are applicable to other mental hospitals and in some ways to general hospital situations. The nurse can evaluate for herself the extent to which our approach is applicable in her own particular nursing situation.

We have disguised all case material to protect the identity of patients and staff. The term "nurse" is used in this book to refer to persons who carry on interpersonal relations with patients and who are responsible for their daily care. Therefore, the terms "attendant," "nurse," "aide," and "student nurse" are used interchangeably.

This book is written for those mental hospital personnel who are in direct and continuous contact with patients. These personnel form emotionally important relationships with patients, make up their social environment, and leave their mark on them for good or ill. Through these relationships personnel can make a significant contribution to an improvement in the patient's living with himself and others. The extent of this contribution has not been measured, nor has it been adequately explored. We hope our book will further this exploration.

In mental hospitals many nurses are doing effective and important work in caring for patients. Though they have been dealing therapeutically with patients for a long time, the knowledge and experience they have developed has not been recorded and organized in such a way that it can be made available to others. The nurse has not been reluctant to share her knowledge and experience, but sometimes she has been unable to explain clearly and precisely what she does that helps the patient, how she does it, why she does it that way, and how she knows when she has been helpful. Frequently she may not know exactly what she does do. She may recognize the activities that are useful for patients but be unable to formulate her thoughts and feelings and describe them either to herself or to others. Or she may be clear about each of her individual actions and relations with patients but not have an adequate framework by which she can organize a wide variety of relations with patients into a coherent picture.

One of our purposes is to make explicit and communicate some of the knowledge and experiences nurses have accumulated. The only way these experiences can be evaluated is to make them widely available for discussion. In the course of doing this, ideas and theories about psychiatric nursing can be examined, tested, modified, and expanded. In the chapters that follow we try to present concretely and specifically much that experienced nurses already know. We also provide a point of view and approach—a scheme of understanding and analysis—with which the nurse can evaluate her experiences. We hope this framework will be useful in helping the nurse clarify and organize her past and present experiences with patients.

We believe that the nurse's job satisfaction and patient improvement are intimately related and develop simultaneously. Thus, another of our purposes is to help the nurse expand her conception of her job and see its potentialities for satisfaction, creative activity, and personal growth. It is difficult, if not impossible, for the nurse to contribute to patient improvement if she is dissatisfied in her job. Stating it another way, the more the nurse helps the patient the greater will be her job satisfaction.

Our intention is not to tell the nurse how she ought to act or how she ought to feel, nor to prescribe specific attitudes she should have or assume, nor to give specific directions as to what she ought to do to get patients well. We cannot, and even if we could, we would not give such specific directives for a number of reasons. First, our knowledge is not precise enough. Second, a procedure that has been useful for one patient may not necessarily be useful for another, and, as a matter of fact, might not be useful for the same patient under different circumstances at another time. Finally, we do not believe a pat formula—a cut-and-dried automatic procedure—will most effectively achieve the nurse's goals. One cannot *order* feelings and attitudes to be *had* by a nurse toward a patient. Such ordering is likely to create resistance on the part of the nurse, to force the nurse to pretend she has the attitudes and feelings ordered, or to lead her to deceive herself (and perhaps the person in authority, but not the patient) into believing she has those feelings and attitudes. Rather, we believe that a general approach that encourages an inquiring and curious attitude and the exploration of different ways of relating to patients will provide the conditions under which the nurse can be most therapeutic. In this book we raise questions that need to be explored in nursing the mentally ill. We try to stimulate thinking about alternative ways of dealing with patients, and we share our experiences with the nurse in order that we may contribute to her solving the problems she meets in her own situations.

In our discussion we focus on one aspect of nursing the mentally ill: the interpersonal relations between patients and nurses. We believe this aspect to be crucial in bringing about patient improvement. Whatever a nurse is doing with the patient— bathing him, feeding him, giving him medication, playing games with him, or sitting and talking with him—she is maintaining a relationship with him. We need to know more about these nurse-patient interactions and to understand their effects on patients. We also focus on the nurse's relations with her colleagues as they affect the patient.

We have omitted from our discussion the ways in which these interpersonal relations are affected by the social organization of the hospital, that is, the ways in which the social context influences and shapes the relations between patients and personnel. However, by this omission we do not mean to leave the impression that we minimize or underestimate the importance of the social context in contributing to or limiting the nurse's therapeutic effectiveness. But the analysis of the social organization of the mental hospital and its therapeutic or nontherapeutic effects would require a book in itself. It has been considered of sufficient importance to be the subject of a recent publication.[1]

We have organized the book in two parts. Part I deals with selected types of problem situations that recur in caring for mental patients. We examine these situations by using specific examples, discussing them, and describing the nurse's and the patient's part in them. In Part II we discuss how the nurse communicates and relates with the patient and the ways in which she might develop a better understanding of him and more appropriate behavior with him.

The relations between staff members, between patients and personnel, and the relations of patients to each other have an important effect on every patient. Throughout the volume we try to contribute to the nurse's awareness and understanding of the subtle and complex ways these relations either facilitate or hinder the patient's improvement.

Perhaps the book can best be used in small discussion groups led by psychiatric nursing educators, supervisors, head nurses, or psychiatrists who are interested in training psychiatric nursing personnel. In such groups, personnel who have the greatest amount of contact with patients can discuss their experiences, compare them with the experiences we present, and evaluate the usefulness of our approach in understanding their relations with patients in their own nursing situations.

The research project that provided most of the data and case materials was entitled "An Investigation to Determine the Modes of Intervention and Social Structure Which Will Facilitate the Recovery of Patients on a Disturbed Ward of a Mental Hospital."

[1] For an extensive discussion of the mental hospital context, see Stanton, A. H., and M. S. Schwartz, *The Mental Hospital*, Basic Books, New York, 1954.

It was supported by a grant (M 493) to the Washington School of Psychiatry by the United States Public Health Service. Additional support for the preparation of this volume was provided by Russell Sage Foundation.

We are indebted to Chestnut Lodge, Inc., for the opportunity to conduct the research. We are particularly grateful to the persons who participated actively in the study: Elizabeth Cline, R.N., Mabel B. Cohen, M.D., Maryan Desmarais, R.N., Bert Harrell, R.N., Norman Rintz, M.D., and Otto A. Will, Jr., M.D., of the hospital staff, and Gwen Tudor Will, R.N., of the United States Public Health Service.

We would like to thank the Washington School of Psychiatry for its administrative assistance. We are especially grateful for the encouragement and support we received from Leonard S. Cottrell, Jr., Ph.D., and Esther Lucile Brown, Ph.D., of Russell Sage Foundation.

Jane Tuttrup was of invaluable assistance in many phases of our work and played a continuing and important role in bringing the book to completion. She searched the records, extracted and helped organize the examples, helped in the revision and editing of the manuscript, and developed the index. Isabel Winner contributed her secretarial skills to the project, and Sylvia Goodstein gave us part-time assistance in typing the manuscript.

In addition to Dr. Brown and Dr. Cottrell, the following persons read the manuscript before publication: Elizabeth S. Bixler, R.N., Dexter M. Bullard, M.D., Joan Cardon, R.N., Marcella Zaleski Davis, R.N., Theresa Fernandez, R.N., Florence Harvey, R.N., Jay Hoffman, M.D., and Eleanor Lewis, R.N. We are indebted to them for their comments, criticisms, and suggestions. Special mention should be made of the editorial work done by Margaret R. Dunne of Russell Sage Foundation in the final preparation of the manuscript.

Charlotte Green Schwartz contributed in many significant ways to the content, the form, and the meaningfulness of the book. The appearance of her name on the title page is insufficient recognition of the debt we owe her.

PART I
RECURRING PROBLEM SITUATIONS

« 1 »

Fear and Patient Assaultiveness

IN the course of her daily activities, a nurse is continually forming relationships with patients, whether she is helping them in
the routines of living, talking casually with them, or trying to ease
the pain and anxiety they are experiencing. Because patients are
mentally ill they have many difficulties in living, and the nurse
who cares for them will have to deal with these difficulties. For
example, when mentally ill patients become assaultive, demanding, or incontinent the nurse has to do something about their
behavior. She has to handle it in some way and many problem
situations arise. In Part I we focus on these problem situations in
order to help the nurse cope with them. We believe that the nurse
can find her own solutions if she is willing to look squarely at
these problem situations and to deal directly with them despite
the discomfort she may have to endure.

One such problem situation that the nurse commonly deals
with is assaultiveness of patients and her own fear of such behavior. It is a rare nurse, indeed, who has not experienced some
fear while working with mental patients, and it is not unusual for
a nurse to be attacked by a patient sometime in the course of her
nursing career. If the nurse can gain some understanding of the
reasons for patient assaultiveness and of her own fear, she may be
able to handle this problem situation more adequately.

Although it is possible to distinguish between fear and anxiety
—in the former the person is afraid of someone or something
concrete that he can point to as the object of his fear, and in the
latter the person feels uneasy about or dreads something he cannot specify—for our purposes we shall not make such refinements.
If the situation is one in which a reaction on the part of a nurse

or patient appears to be what we ordinarily call fear, we shall treat it as fear. We do this because nurses generally use the word "fear" to refer to both fear and anxiety; many of these situations of fear are a mixture of both, and it would be difficult to discriminate between them in each situation.

THE NURSE IS AFRAID

There are various processes that contribute initially to the nurse's fear of patients and that subsequently help to maintain this fear. We can begin to identify these by describing three general *sources* of the nurse's fear: (a) her own preconceptions, expectations, and feelings, (b) the activities and attitudes of the group with which she works, and (c) the activities and attitudes of patients with whom she works.

The Nurse's Preconceptions, Expectations, and Feelings

Even though they have never seen any mental patients, many people are afraid of "them." Mental patients are thought to be peculiar and unconventional; associated with this thought is the idea that they are impulsive and frequently attack others. The stereotype of the mentally ill person is the "homicidal maniac" whom one should avoid. Nurses share this *cultural stereotype* that mental patients are assaultive and dangerous. If the nurse can see the preconception as an idea that heretofore she has taken for granted and that may have little foundation in fact, she may be able to reduce her fear of patients.

The way a nurse's expectations may be related to patient assaultiveness in the hospital is shown in the following example:

A nurse came to work in a mental hospital, bringing with her from another hospital the idea that patients became assaultive and blew up at the "full of the moon." Up to the time of her arrival no one had noticed any particular connection between excessive outbreaks of violence and a full moon. A short while after the nurse's arrival, this idea spread among hospital personnel. At the next full moon there was a noticeable increase in violence. The following month, prior to the full moon, nursing personnel talked about the expected attacks and the difficult time they were going to have with patients' assaults at the full of the moon. Again, there was an increased amount of violence at that time. This continued for six months. Each month the nurses dreaded the full moon and expected patients to become violent, and each time they did. By this time personnel were convinced of the inevitability of these outbreaks. One nurse, however, questioned their inevitability, saying that the idea was a myth. Other nurses pointed out to her that violence did in fact increase at these times. The nurse, in turn, claimed that the attacks were due to their fear and anticipation of them. She was able to convince many nurses that if they could relax and not expect the attacks at the full of the moon, these outbreaks might not happen. At the next full moon there was much less discussion and mutual stimulation of fear and anticipation, and the assaultiveness was no greater than at any other time of the month. Nor did assaultiveness recur subsequently to any greater degree at the full of the moon.

In the foregoing illustration the nurses' *expectation* of assaults at a certain time seemed to play an important part in bringing them about. Personnel approached the patients with a great deal of fear, expecting to be attacked at the time of the full moon. The nurses' fear and expectation of attack seemed to encourage and stimulate the patients' assaultiveness.

There are many ways in which the nurse's expectations increase her fear of a patient. Some recognition of the ways in which these fears develop, how they get established, and what they are based on may help her to understand and cope with them. In the conference that follows, nurses and aides are discussing their fear of a patient, Mrs. Reed.

MISS JONES: I was scared of Mrs. Reed the first time I saw her, before anybody said anything about her. But I think, too, I continued to be afraid of her because nobody would go in her room. And I was waiting to see if somebody would go in.

SOCIOLOGIST: Maybe you have some experiences you'd like to talk about. Why are we so afraid? What's behind this whole business of fear?

MRS. RUSH: I think people are afraid because nobody likes to be hurt.

SOCIOLOGIST: Do you believe you'll be hurt seriously by any of the patients?

MISS TRENT: You *can* be hurt or injured.

SOCIOLOGIST: Has anybody that you know of been injured by these patients?

MRS. RUSH: I don't know about here. I've read all my life about people in mental hospitals. You hear about all these things and when you get there you never see any evidence of them.

MISS JONES: I think it's not knowing what the patient might do, more than the actual blows. It's like when I was standing next to Sally on the porch one day. I think I was more scared waiting for her to do something than if she had gone ahead and hit me. If we had put her in her room and got it over with, that wouldn't have been so bad as just standing there. It seems I stood there for an awfully long time.

MISS TRENT: The anticipation is worse than anything else.

MISS JONES: I think the preconceived notions we have about mental hospitals diminish after we have been here awhile.

MISS TRENT: I was in a situation where a woman beat the tar out of me, but until that happened I was afraid of its happening, and after it happened I wasn't scared of her any longer.

MISS JONES: I think after you're hit the first time you don't mind it so much. You are afraid—"Gosh, she's going to hit me,"—and you don't know what's going to happen. The time Mrs. Reed hit me I was dazed for a little while, but I found I still had my head. . . . Now I think if she would hit me again I wouldn't mind so much. As it was, she did it so fast that I didn't know what was happening. Now I don't tremble. All my fear isn't gone, but I feel better about it.

SOCIOLOGIST: Having experienced it, you find that the experience is never so bad as the anticipation.

MISS JONES: It hasn't bothered me since the first time I was hit, and I don't get banged up so much now either.

SOCIOLOGIST: The less fear you show, the less possibility there will be of your getting hit. These patients are not hitting you because they want to frighten you. They're hitting you because they're so frightened themselves. They hit in self-defense.

MISS TRENT: I think I can honestly say that when I never thought I was going to be hit I never have been. I've been swung at and missed sometimes.

MISS JONES: I think part of our fear is that we just don't like to be hit and we don't like to be pushed around.

SOCIOLOGIST: It hurts your self-esteem somewhat? I wonder if there's more to fear than just physical fear.

MRS. RUSH: Maybe you don't like to be rejected.

MISS JONES: Maybe it's because you're afraid of your own anger and that you'll hit back. It's been ingrained in us that one should not hit these patients, that they're not responsible. Everybody said that was the right attitude, and I kept thinking if I got hit, I might hit back.

SOCIOLOGIST: You think that means there's something wrong with you. Everybody is supposed to accept this and you can't—you might hit back. Is part of the difficulty that you don't want to think of yourself as being so brutal? Everybody else supposedly can restrain himself and you can't. Isn't there a difference between impulsive anger and deliberate cruelty?

MISS JONES: There's something else tied up with this. Whenever a patient gets assaultive with us, we're concerned with what the other personnel are going to think. They might think that we did something to bring it about.

SOCIOLOGIST: You mean that if a patient hits you, you have failed; that if you had conducted yourself differently it would not have occurred.

MISS JONES: You have the feeling that you have upset the patient, and other people will think so too.

There are several points made above that are worth highlighting. Sometimes a nurse brings her anticipation of attack and fear of a patient to the ward with her, and her fear is reinforced when she sees other personnel avoiding a patient because they, too, are fearful. At times, the anticipation of attack creates more fear than the actual attack. The nurse is not only afraid of being hurt; *she is also afraid of being rejected, afraid of her own anger and desire to hit back, and afraid of her colleagues' disapproval.* Often nurses have a difficult time recognizing that they are afraid, and even after they do see their fear, they are reluctant to admit it to others. A nurse may feel she must pretend she is not afraid because "nurses are not supposed to be afraid," and this need to deny her fear may be encouraged by her fellow workers. This attitude of denial and need to put up a brave front is not helpful to the nurse. Admitting the fear to oneself and being able to talk about it with others appears to be a necessary first step to understanding and reducing it. Nurses may also have a difficult time recognizing that they feel hostile toward the patient. If they are aware of hostile feelings, they may be afraid that they will not be able to control their impulses to retaliate. Here, too, a recognition of their feelings might help them handle them more adequately.

Another type of preconception and expectation, which is not ordinarily thought of as such, is the *patient's reputation.* When a patient has a certain reputation among nurses it means, in effect, that nurses expect certain things from him and anticipate a particular kind of relationship with him. In the situation described below we see how a patient's reputation is spread.

> Miss Jones, a nurse who had not worked on the Fifth Ward, had been talking about Mr. Smith to various people who had worked there. The patient had been assaultive in the past, but recently had not assaulted anyone. Nevertheless, ward personnel were still afraid of him, and his reputation as a "dangerous" patient persisted and was conveyed to Miss Jones. When she was questioned about working on that ward, she replied, "I would enjoy it up there, but I am too terrified of Mr. Smith, and yet I have never had any contact with him."

At times nurses do not realize that their fear of a patient may not be justified—that the patient does not deserve the reputation he has. Because he was assaultive in the past, personnel believe he will be assaultive in the future. They convey their fear to each other and to new personnel who come to the ward. In this way the patient's reputation as an assaultive person becomes standardized and reinforced. In this way, too, personnel might help to bring about the very assaults that convince them that the patient's reputation is justified.

When a nurse is not aware of a patient's reputation she may be able to deal with him in terms of *her own experience* with him, and not rely exclusively on the experience of others.

> A patient, Mr. Holmes, had the reputation of attacking without warning, and because of this was in seclusion much of the time. Personnel would enter his room with extreme caution and no more frequently than necessary. The patient was generally avoided, and personnel expressed their fear quite openly. One day a new student nurse, who was not acquainted with the patient's reputation, unlocked his door and spent a half hour chatting with him. She later related her experience to the regular ward personnel, who became quite alarmed. They told the student about the patient's past behavior and indicated that it was unwise to be in the room alone with him. After this talk the student, too, became frightened. She was reluctant to visit with the patient and adopted the staff's attitude of caution and avoidance.

The significant point in this example is the contrast in the student's attitude and behavior. When she was unaware of the patient's reputation and had no preconceptions about him, she acted spontaneously and could visit with him without fear and without being attacked. As soon as the others communicated their fear and the patient's reputation to her, and *despite her own pleasant experience with the patient*, she, too, became afraid of him.

We have suggested that there is a connection between the nurse's expectations, preconceptions, and feelings and the patient's assaultiveness. We have said that often the nurse's expectation of assault and her fear of the patient tend to bring about the very attack she fears. By approaching the patient in a frightened manner or by avoiding him because of fear, the personnel seem to "provoke" or "invite" him to attack them. It seems that by these expectations the nurse conveys the attitude that the patient is a person to be feared, that he is dangerous and terrible. The patient has this attitude toward himself. Thus, the nurse reinforces the patient's conceptions of himself as a dangerous person by also having that attitude toward him. When the patient looks upon himself as a dangerous person he then *has to* act as such by assaulting others. In this way the nurse, at least in part, tends to perpetuate the patient's attacks. If this interpretation is correct, a change in the nurse's attitudes toward the patient and expectations of him may change his assaultive behavior, because she may help him change his conception of himself as a violent person.

One way in which the nurse might develop some perspective on her fear and perhaps reduce it is to assume a questioning attitude toward a patient's reputation. As an aid to developing a more realistic and broader view we suggest that the nurse try to answer the following questions about an assaultive patient:

   1. Can you identify the preconceptions, expectations, and feelings you have about this patient? In order to do something about her attitudes and feelings the nurse has to be aware of them.
   2. Do you know where and how you acquired these expectations? Did they come from other people's reports about the patient, or from your experience with him? If the nurse discovers that she does not

know how she developed her expectations, she might be interested in reexamining them and questioning their validity.

3. Is your feeling about the patient based on one incident or on a number of assaults that form a consistent picture?

4. Are you afraid of the patient? Is it physical injury that you fear, or something else?

5. If you are afraid of a patient, are there others who are not? If the nurse can discover the reasons for another's lack of fear, she might be able to discover how to change her own fear.

6. Does the patient deserve the reputation he has? Has he really hurt someone? When was the last time he attacked anyone? What portion of the day or week does he spend in hostile attack? By actually counting the assaults the nurse might be able to make a realistic appraisal of how dangerous the patient really is.

7. Have there been times when the patient might have been assaultive and was not? Are you overlooking these situations and concentrating on his attacks? Have there been times when this patient was pleasant and friendly? Can you find the reasons for this difference in behavior?

8. With whom and when is the patient assaultive? What are some of the reasons for this? If the nurse can ask herself questions about the circumstances under which the patient becomes hostile and attacks, she might be able to prevent the attack.

9. With whom is he rarely or never assaultive? What are the reasons for this? If the nurse can discover the kind of relationship with the patient that makes it unnecessary for him to be assaultive, she can then work toward establishing that kind of relationship.

10. Have you or any of the other personnel ever changed your attitude toward an assaultive patient? If so, under what circumstances and with what results? What helped to bring about the change in attitude?

The Group's Contribution to the Nurse's Fear

Since the nursing situation is always a group situation, it is inevitable that nurses will influence each other's attitudes, opinions, and feelings about patients. This is especially true when they discuss their fear of a patient. There are many ways in which her group helps the nurse understand and reduce her fear and gives her support and encouragement. But it is also from her group that she may acquire, maintain, and reinforce her fear of a patient and her expectation that he will be assaultive. Here we will look at the way in which the group contributes to the nurse's fear. In the next chapter we will indicate how the group can help her handle her fear.

In the following example a graduate nurse reports on the origin of a student nurse's fear.

> MRS. PRATT: Do you remember when we were talking about Sheryl Smith's [student nurse] fear and how it started? She told me that personnel were talking about Mrs. Reed's being assaultive and their being afraid of her, and this made her afraid. She had spent a lot of time with Mrs. Reed on Seventh [another ward], and she used to enjoy being with her. But when Mrs. Reed got upset and came down here [to the disturbed ward] Sheryl would listen to the personnel telling how assaultive she could be and about some of the things she was doing, and this made her afraid of Mrs. Reed. She thought that Mrs. Reed must be pretty hard to manage because Mr. Quinn [an aide] was staying with her all the time and was the only one having any contact with her.

In this illustration the student nurse's fear is built up by hearing the group talk about their fear—talk that concentrates on and emphasizes their fear and the patient's assaultiveness. We have said before that talking openly about her fear may be useful in helping the nurse cope with it. However, open discussion is only the first step. In itself it does not ensure that the nurse will be helped to handle her fear. If the discussion consists mainly of accounts of assaultive incidents, expressions of fear, and warnings to keep away from the patient, it may only reinforce the nurse's fear and make it difficult for her to approach the patient. One way of evaluating the usefulness of such a discussion is to analyze it in terms of its purpose, the direction it is taking, its content, its effects, and the attitudes of the participants during the discussion. If these discussions have constructive elements, they will emphasize the signs the patient gives of a forthcoming attack; what can be done to calm the patient or prevent the attack; and how the attack might be dealt with, once it has occurred. Knowledge about an assaultive patient gained from working with him over a considerable length of time can be useful to a new nurse if it is communicated to her without focusing exclusively on the fear of the patient.

The conference of sociologist, nurses, aides, and students that follows illustrates some effects of the group upon the attitudes and feelings of nursing personnel.

SOCIOLOGIST: Have you noticed any subtle ways in which you adopt the attitudes of other personnel, and lo and behold you wake up one day and you have their attitudes?

MISS JONES [a student nurse]: Well I think the attitudes toward Sam Jackson are sort of catching. Everybody seems to steer clear of him.

SOCIOLOGIST: Why don't you talk about that a little bit? I think it would be interesting.

MISS JONES: I really don't know what to say. Every time you go into his room he says, "Excuse me, please," and sometimes he says it very belligerently. You just take it that he wants you to get out, so we do. You know we've been doing that. Since the time he hit the student I've been afraid to go in there. We've all been afraid to go in there. He's pretty frightening, you know.

SOCIOLOGIST: You think everybody feels the same way?

MISS JONES: I heard people saying they were scared, and nobody goes in there unless he has to.

MISS HARDY: There is hardly anybody who would go into his room.

SOCIOLOGIST: What frightened you besides the student's getting hit?

MISS JONES: I don't know, but he scared me even before I knew his name. He was so big and looked rather wild.

SOCIOLOGIST: So you were frightened by him. He kept saying, "Excuse me," and everyone thinks that means, "Get out of here or I'll bop you one," so they leave quickly.

MISS JONES: Mr. Kelly [an aide] goes in there almost every day. I think he's the only one that really spends any time with him.

MISS HARDY: I don't think he spends too much time, but some nearly every day.

SOCIOLOGIST: He goes in, anyway.

MISS HARDY: Yes, and he stays.

SOCIOLOGIST: So there's at least one person who seems not to be so afraid of him. Well, the thing I would like you to think about is the fact that each of you fears him. You really haven't had much experience with him, yet you're afraid. How come?

MISS JONES: This fear gets communicated.

SOCIOLOGIST: Other personnel communicate it to you and vice versa.

MRS. ADAMS: Well, two people always take a tray to him. It makes me more afraid of him when I see that it takes two people to bring him his tray.

SOCIOLOGIST: You show each other you are frightened and you reinforce it by keeping away from the patient yourself, as well as seeing others keep away from him.

MRS. KING: People on the ward tell us how assaultive he used to be, even though he may not be that way today.

SOCIOLOGIST: That is, his past determines your present attitude toward him. We used to be children once, you know, and we don't treat each other as if we still were.

MRS. ADAMS: People on the ward seem to try to convince you how assaultive he is, and that you should keep away from him.

SOCIOLOGIST: I wonder why they try to convince you. It would seem that the opposite would be more useful. He breaks out every once in a while, but 99 per cent of the time he's all right. Why do you think people have to convince you that he's so dangerous?

MISS JONES: I don't know, but it didn't occur to me to think about it. Now I find I'm asking if he really is so assaultive.

SOCIOLOGIST: That's a good question to ask.

MRS. KING: People really try to scare you.

SOCIOLOGIST: Well why do you think personnel try to convince you the patient is so assaultive? They're not being nasty and trying to frighten you, are they?

MRS. KING: I don't think so.

SOCIOLOGIST: Well, what is the reason?

MRS. ADAMS: They want to protect you.

SOCIOLOGIST: Do you think that's their only motive—to protect you?

MISS JONES: Maybe they want us to be frightened so they'll have company; then they won't feel so bad.

MISS BAKER: If you say this is an assaultive patient, then you don't have any responsibility for behaving differently toward the patient—for taking care of him.

SOCIOLOGIST: Might it be that if you yourself are frightened, then it's rather hard to think that you are frightened and other people may not be, and that there's something wrong with you. Whereas if you're frightened and other people are frightened, too, there's nothing wrong with you—everything is wrong with the patient. So if you get everybody feeling the same way about this patient, it makes it easier on you. People don't like to feel fear. It's a little more comfortable to feel it if everybody else does. Then you aren't so cowardly.

MISS BAKER: Human beings want to share their feelings about fear. This might be one way one shares it with somebody else—to make him feel a little of it.

SOCIOLOGIST: In terms of being more useful to the patient, it might be of much more use to say, "He got upset and assaultive and I was kind of scared, but I got over it,"—if you did.

MRS. ADAMS: I sure had a hard time going back after Dr. James said he was scared of Mr. Jackson, too.

MISS JONES: Carol [a student nurse who had been successful with patients] said that the way to get over fear is to spend more time with the patient.

MISS BAKER: And know more about him. Do the things that he'll accept and you get to feeling better about him. Then you don't have to get so scared.

SOCIOLOGIST: So much of this talk tends to keep us away rather than to help us spend more time with patients. If the patient hasn't been assaultive for a long, long time and suddenly breaks out for a little while, it's so easy to change your attitude and label the patient "assaultive" even though much of the time he hasn't been so; and it's not easy to change back.

MRS. ADAMS: When you talk about your fear this way with others you're not even aware of what you're doing. If you become aware of it you might be able to stop it. It certainly doesn't help you if you inspire somebody else with fear. What he is going to do is come back next time and do the same thing to you. You might get over it if somebody didn't reinforce it in you.

MISS HARDY: It's a very powerful thing that happens if a patient inspires you with fear. It collects and collects until the patient can no longer function on the ward. And the same stories are passed from ward to ward so that he can no longer function in the hospital.

SOCIOLOGIST: I think the important thing to remember is that if you're so fearful, you're going to arouse the same fear in the patient, and that's why you might get hit—you solicit it. The patient usually is aware of your fear and that you're in effect saying to him, "You're such a frightening creature." After all, it only stimulates his anxiety and about the only outlet he has is to be a frightening creature.

MISS BAKER: If a patient once becomes assaultive, it is much easier for him to remain assaultive because he's got the reputation of being assaultive. When he stops, everybody's still expecting it and no one treats him in a completely relaxed way.

SOCIOLOGIST: In other words the patient fits into what your attitude is toward him, which attitude in the first place he helped to create and you also helped to establish. So it goes round and round in a cycle.

MISS BAKER: It's self-perpetuating.

SOCIOLOGIST: That's a good observation. If you can catch up with these attitudes you can do something about them.

This conference demonstrates that group members can play an important part in either perpetuating the nurse's fear or in helping her understand and lessen her fear. Greater freedom from fear can be developed in the group if the members are curious about their own fear and how it affects the patient. The discussion can be directed, as it was by the sociologist, toward finding out what the nurse's fear is, what it is based on, how it is communicated, what motivations there are in communicating it, what it means to the nurse, and what effects it has.

The reports of nurses to each other at change of shifts are a group activity that may contribute to or diminish a nurse's fear of a patient. If the reporting nurse focuses on the patient's assaultiveness and omits mention of his other activities, she, quite unconsciously, may give the impression that the patient's assaultiveness was much greater than it actually was. She may also leave the oncoming personnel with the anticipation that the patient will be assaultive. If, however, the patient's assaultiveness is placed in the context of his other activities and the nurse gives a full report, the oncoming personnel may have a less biased perspective. Patients are seldom continuously assaultive or as "violent" as a selective report might represent them to be. If, day after day, only the patient's assaults are described, the group may stabilize an attitude of fear and an expectation of assault from the patient that may be hard to change.

Our final illustration of the contribution of the group to a nurse's fear shows the effects of extreme fear. A patient, Mrs. Patterson, had been assaultive for the past month, and personnel became increasingly fearful of her, until something like a "wall of fear" had been built around her. Personnel were cautious, tended to avoid her, visited her only when necessary and then only when another person was along. When someone entered the room, the patient often attacked, and personnel entered expecting attack. In addition, the patient was secluded a good deal of the time. When let out of seclusion, she attacked people and had to be taken to her room after a short while. Personnel usually talked about these attacks and their fear of the patient and indicated their desire to keep away from her because she was so dangerous.

One experienced nurse, Miss Nixon, who was less frightened of the patient than other personnel, describes the results of the widespread fear of this patient.

MISS NIXON: Miss Jackson [an aide] came running up to me and said, "Come help me! Mrs. Patterson is going to attack Mr. Smith [another patient]!" Miss Jackson didn't try to do anything about it; she just ran to me for help. When I went to get Mrs. Patterson away from Mr. Smith she grabbed me by the arm and started to bite me. I tried to get away and yelled for help. Miss Jackson backed clear down the hall, too scared to come near me; a student was just frozen. I saw Miss Niles [an aide] go into Stella's [a patient's] room. I think she saw what was going on but ducked into the room. I kept yelling, "Somebody help me!" but nobody did. Everyone just stood there.
SOCIOLOGIST: Nobody came to your help?
MISS NIXON: Nobody at all. When I asked Miss Niles about it she said she "didn't know what to do." When I asked Miss Jackson, "Why didn't you help me? Why were you standing there? I wouldn't stand there when you were getting bitten!"—she said, "I didn't know what I could do." But Miss Jackson is so terrified of patients that I can scarcely get her out of the office. She won't talk about her fear. She says she's not afraid, but she resists coming to work. She's good about making beds and cleaning up, and so I try to use her in that capacity.
SOCIOLOGIST: It seems that's what she wants.
MISS NIXON: She runs into the office every possible minute. If Mrs. Patterson begins yelling, she won't go into her room. She'll run into the linen closet. She just runs her legs off keeping away. If Mrs. Board [a patient] or Sally [another patient] is yelling, she also stays away from them.
SOCIOLOGIST: How about Miss Cantor [a nurse]? Where was she?
MISS NIXON: She said she didn't see it, but whenever Mrs. Patterson gets upset she never rushes out to help. They were all afraid, but I sure was mad that nobody came to help me. After I had calmed down and had time to think, it came to me—no wonder everybody is so afraid of Mrs. Patterson. They are scared to death that if they get into a struggle with her nobody will come to their help. While I was angry I thought about other hospitals I've worked in. We always felt that when someone else got hurt by a patient it was our fault because we weren't there to help.
SOCIOLOGIST: You feel that you would want to help someone else, and it's important to know that someone will help you, that she wants to help you.
MISS NIXON: I was upset about being attacked, but I was also upset that I couldn't rely on anybody to help me.

Once the ward personnel have developed such an intense and widespread fear of a patient, it is difficult for a particular nurse not to be fearful. This fear may come to include other patients, even though there may not be much reason to be afraid of them. Such extreme fear on the part of a nurse, when shared by other personnel, can become demoralizing to the group as a whole. Group support is an important factor in dealing with assaultive patients. If this is not forthcoming, one nurse will be reluctant to help another nurse, first, because she is afraid and, second, because no one comes to help her when she is attacked. In this way, fear of personnel and inadequate handling of the patient are perpetuated.

The Patient's Contribution to the Nurse's Fear

Not only does the nurse's fear arise from her own and the group's expectations, but the feelings and activities of the patients also contribute to it. For the fact of the matter is that some patients do make threatening gestures, some do attack and seriously hurt people, and some do present themselves as persons to be feared. What the nurse has to determine is the appropriateness of her fear to the real situation. Is the nurse's fear more or less than the patient's actual or potential assaultiveness warrants; that is, is it realistic and appropriate to the danger in the situation? Once the nurse puts her fear into proper perspective, she may be less restricted and less limited in her thinking and be able to devise ways of coping with it and of protecting herself against injury in a way that might also be useful to the patient.

There are a number of things a nurse finds hard to accept in regard to assaultiveness, other than the possibility of physical injury or pain. A patient's attack may appear highly irrational. In the past the nurse might have had a good relation with the patient, or she may have been trying to help him when the attack occurred. Thus, the attack is not understandable, and she feels hurt because she feels she has been trying to help the patient and has not done anything to provoke or deserve the attack. Under these circumstances, it is difficult for her to realize that the patient may be seeing her as someone else and thinks he is attacking that other person. The patient may not feel hostile toward the nurse herself but it is difficult for nurses not to take these attacks personally. In addition to the irrationality of the attack, its suddenness, its unpredictability, its variability, and the fact that it alternates with friendly behavior, all may make it difficult for the nurse to understand it.

In the illustration given below the sociologist is relating his experience with a patient and trying to find out some of the factors that made him fearful in this situation.

SOCIOLOGIST: I want to tell you about what happened with Belle Duncan yesterday. I went up to the living room, and she was walking around there, and I said, "Hi," and she said, "Hello." At first she was friendly, then a whole series of things happened very quickly. She started raving at me, not so much in words, but just shouting in a very hoarse voice. She did that for a few minutes with both of us standing by the door. Finally I said, "Sit down." And she said, "Oh, do you want to sit down?" So then I went and sat down and she just stood. And every time I looked at her she would get terribly frightened, and start to rage, with more of this bellowing. And if I made a move she would hold a finger over me and say, "Stop! Don't move!" She had a very wild look in her eyes. And at one point she just stamped her foot so hard I thought she would break the floor and my ears. I said, "Belle, you are hurting my ears," and she stopped. I got very frightened when she held her hands up as if she was going to claw me, and she came close. At another point she put her fist up and drew it back. But that didn't make me so frightened as when she started to bellow, as if she was just trying to tear her guts out. It was animal-like and terrifying. I got some very nice support from the people there; Miss Blaine [a nurse] sat right by the door in a chair, and I could see her all the time, so I knew she was there. Miss Cressy [a nurse] was there, and also a student. Their being around was quite reassuring. So the fear sort of subsided after a while, and I decided the only thing to do was just to sit there and not look at her. If I even glanced at her she would shake and tremble and get much more anxious and hoarse, and shout. . . . And I tried not to move because when I did she'd have to put up her finger and say, "Hold it." I wasn't afraid she was going to hurt me, but when she shouted, I got terribly frightened. That disturbed me very much. Then toward the end she walked around and lowered her voice and started to sob. At the end she walked by very gracefully, away from the door.

The thing that quite impressed me was this up and down business. Now you are on and now you are off; now you are my friend and now you are my enemy. In other words, you never get any kind of stability. You can't tell what will happen in your relationship with her. There's no continuity from one day to the next, or from one hour to the next. You don't know what she is going to do, and you don't know what to expect. Also, you don't know who she thinks you are. And this, I think, is probably one of the most difficult things for us to take.

Not knowing what to expect from the patient nor how to act toward her, contributed to the sociologist's fear. There did not seem to be enough stability in his relationship with the patient to permit him to be comfortable with her in this difficult situation. However, at times a patient's attack is sufficiently understood by the nurse, despite its apparent irrationality, that she can try to discuss the situation with the patient and work it out with him.

A nurse is talking about a patient, Miss Conway.

MISS ALLEN: Miss Conway hit me in the nose today. I tried to stop her from getting out the door. I grabbed hold of her, and she hit me. John and Dell [personnel] were right there, but neither one of them came near me.

SOCIOLOGIST: Nobody came to your help?

MISS ALLEN: No. Miss Conway went back to her room screaming for me at the top of her lungs. So I went back. She screamed, "You're a thief! You're a liar! You've stolen my belt!" She was crying and was upset. So I opened her bureau drawer and found her belt. She had a regular temper tantrum right after she hit me.

SOCIOLOGIST: What do you think that meant?

MISS ALLEN: I think she was very upset for having hit me.

SOCIOLOGIST: Did you have a chance to talk with her about it?

MISS ALLEN: The next morning I said to her, "I don't think you were really mad at me. I wish you'd figure out whom you want to hit in the nose. I would sure like to know what's wrong." She said, "I'm sleeping, don't bother me." So we didn't talk much. This thing about her going back to her room and screaming about her belt—I think she wanted to see if I'd come back.

SOCIOLOGIST: It is the same with Mrs. Board. After she hits you she gets friendly, because she wants to make sure you haven't abandoned her.

MISS ALLEN: Miss Conway was really in panic afterward.

SOCIOLOGIST: Did you find out anything about it?

MISS ALLEN: I didn't feel she was mad at me when she did it, and I found out later another patient had hit her.

SOCIOLOGIST: So you didn't have to react personally.

MISS ALLEN: I was sure she wasn't mad at me. I found out that after the other patient hit her, she jumped up and down and screamed, "They're attacking me. I've been killed!" She was panicky.

SOCIOLOGIST: She shows us how really frightened she is.

It is important to see that the patient is assaultive for a reason. Sometimes the reason is related primarily to his fantastic thoughts or irrational feelings; at other times it is related to his participation with those around him. Frequently it involves both. The nurse's job is to discover those aspects of her relationship with the patient that encourage or provoke him to be assaultive and contribute to her fear. When she can do this, she is ready to ask herself what she can do to change the situation.

The Effects of the Nurse's Fear on Her Relations with Patients

What are some of the effects of the nurse's fear on her relations with patients? We pointed out previously that her fear might contribute to the continuation of the patient's assaultiveness. This happens if the nurse's fear stimulates the patient to be assaultive. The assaults might continue if a stable situation is established in which the patient's assaults stimulate the nurse's fear and her fear, in turn, helps to bring about the assaults.

Another effect of the nurse's fear is that it prevents her from thinking clearly about the situation, her relationship with the patient, and how to change it. The experience of fear has a way of blurring her ability to think and produces an impulse to run from the situation. This desire and tendency to avoid the patient can have several effects. It may result in neglect of the patient and make for difficulties in being useful to him. As we have seen, the nurse's need to withdraw from the patient is due not only to her fear but also to the fact that she experiences an impulse to retaliate. This impulse is unpleasant to recognize and face, and rather than struggle with it she often prefers to avoid the whole situation. This avoidance and the inability to think clearly about the situation make it difficult for the nurse to set realistic limits for the patient she fears. She may either be unable to "control" him at all because of her fear, or she may become punishing and use the power at her disposal to "keep the patient in line." These extremes do not solve the problem adequately.

Another recourse for the fearful nurse is to seclude and isolate the patient. Such a procedure, if continued for long periods of time, may tend to perpetuate the patient's illness by reinforcing his resentment toward the staff, reinforcing his loneliness and his withdrawal, and strengthening his feeling that other persons are not concerned with his welfare but rather with hurting and punishing him. In some cases because of her fear, the nurse may develop a strong dislike for and distrust of a patient, so that even when he is quiet she may be suspicious that he will attack at any moment. Such feelings make it difficult for the nurse to act spontaneously with the patient and tend to perpetuate mutual distance and strain. Finally, the nurse's fear blocks her from seeing the patient's own fears and insecurities. The more she becomes preoccupied with her own fear, the less she is able to see how frightened the patient is and to figure out ways of relieving his fear.

The Patient Is Afraid

After a nurse has worked in a mental hospital for a short while she realizes how frightened many of the patients are. When she looks for the reasons for a patient's fear she finds at least two: (1) his cultural stereotype of what the mental hospital is like, and (2) his attitudes and feelings about people in general. The patient, like other people, has acquired some of the common attitudes about the mental hospital. It is thought to be a place where patients will be abused, injured, or mistreated. This attitude derives from the past when patients were kept in chains, and also from exposés that have appeared in newspapers from time to time dramatically portraying the brutality or neglect patients experience in a mental hospital. Whether or not the patient fears physical injury by the staff, he may fear that he will be attacked by other patients. This fear and expectation of injury may be maintained despite the fact that he has had few experiences in the hospital that justify it. Such is the strength of these stereotypes and expectations.

The patient may be afraid that "once you're crazy, you'll always be crazy." This means for the patient that he will never get out of the hospital. The expectation that he will have to stay there the rest of his life may fill the patient with dread, and he may express this fear by fighting to get out. The patient may also have a fear of people in general. He may feel that people are not to be trusted, that they are likely to hurt him if he gets too close to them, that they will reject him, or that all one can expect from another person is emotional or physical pain—something he is familiar with from his past experiences. Some of the patient's fears of others—the nurse in the hospital, for example—may be quite irrational. He may misunderstand the nurse's intentions toward him and misinterpret a friendly gesture as a hostile one. At times he may carry his fears to such an extreme that he believes the nurse is going to kill him. The reasons for these misinterpretations and fears may vary from patient to patient, but in general, they have developed from the patient's past experiences in which others have actually been hostile and injurious. While a patient is afraid a nurse is going to hurt him, he may at the same time be struggling with his own impulses to attack her. He may be afraid of these impulses, and especially afraid that he will not be able to control them. He is afraid of himself and what he might do. His fears may also be related to the fantasies he is having at the time, in which he is injuring someone or being injured, or seeing horrible things. Finally, if the patient feels hostile toward the nurse, he may be afraid that the nurse has discovered or will discover these feelings in him and will punish him.

It is sometimes difficult for nurses to understand these fears, especially the terror the patient may at times experience. When a patient is assaultive, the nurse finds it especially difficult to see how frightened he really is, and that he may feel very guilty about what he has done to her. This may be due to the fact that at these times the patient appears so fierce and threatening that he is successful in concealing or disguising his own fear. Or the nurse becomes so preoccupied with her own fear that she is unable to see the patient's fear. In addition, the patient may need to hide his fear from others.

The importance of understanding the patient's fear is stated by a graduate nurse who was at the hospital for a three-month affiliation.

> MISS GREEN: Perhaps the most important thing that happened to me was that I became able to accept the idea that these patients are terribly frightened people. Once I was able to assimilate this, I seemed to gain some freedom to function with these patients. Also, I found it helpful to remember their fright when I was scared to death or so angry, I'd like to have slapped their faces.

In addition to indicating the importance of recognizing the patient's fear, the nurse points out that the patient may be frightened at the same time that the nurse is. Sometimes the nurse and patient are afraid of each other without quite realizing it. What happens is that the nurse conveys her fear to the patient, or the patient communicates his fear to the nurse, and in so doing each reinforces the fear of the other. In this way the patient's fear comes partly from what the nurse does (she shows her fear to him) and the nurse's fear comes partly from what the patient does (he shows his fear to her, and/or becomes assaultive).

We mentioned previously that the patient may be afraid of a nurse for irrational reasons. These irrational sources of his fear can scarcely be controlled by the nurse; the patient's fantasies and emotions develop in many ways and for unknown reasons and cannot be directed according to the nurse's or the patient's wishes. This does not mean, however, that the nurse cannot influence them. For example, the patient may be less terrified by his fantasies if she can reassure him in an appropriate way. But in addition to having these irrational fears, the patient may be afraid because of some real experiences he has had in the hospital, experiences in which one nurse or another has been punitive in action or attitude. Such responses to a patient as cruelty toward him, attacks on him, or retaliation against him tend to perpetuate his fear and may bring about his assaultiveness.

In the following instance a nurse is discussing a patient's assaultiveness with the sociologist. Ordinarily she is not assaultive, and they are trying to understand the reason for her attacks at this time.

> Miss Abel: Miss Conway threw an ashtray at me, and we told her she would have to stay in her room for a while.
>
> Sociologist: I have the feeling that this outbreak of assaultiveness is tied up with some kind of retaliation. One way to increase a patient's assaultiveness is to retaliate for what she does. As soon as you push her around, all she can do is fight back.
>
> Miss Abel: She made me mad. That's why I put her in her room. That's the way I felt I wanted to handle it. I wasn't going to stand there and listen to her filthy language. I made her stay in her room awhile.
>
> Sociologist: Was there any other way of handling it?
>
> Miss Abel: Not at that time. I was mad.
>
> Sociologist: How about after you got over being mad?
>
> Miss Abel: I don't care for her too much.
>
> Sociologist: I think that's interesting. That's how you build up an attitude toward a patient. You have an incident with her, you get angry, and then you have the attitude, "Well, I don't care for her." If you could go back to see her—I'm sure it's difficult while you're still angry—but afterward, go back and talk with her, you might find out why she threw the ashtray, what it is you might have done to annoy her, how you could prevent this in the future. If you try to talk it over with her, I think you wouldn't have to feel that you want to avoid her and that she is somebody you dislike.

Patients are usually very sensitive to the hostile feelings and actions of nurses. When a nurse retaliates against a patient or feels hostile toward him, she can easily stimulate and reinforce his fear.

We have pointed out that fear is easily communicated from patients to personnel and vice versa. Similarly, fear is easily communicated or transferred from one patient to another. When one patient becomes terror-stricken or panicky, this fear is very quickly conveyed to other patients, whose own fears are stimulated. Where patients are living together in a confined physical space, it is easy for one patient to take over the fear of another, especially if this fear is intense and continues for a long period of time.

By and large a patient's fear, if continued for a long period of time, may help to maintain his illness. As a result of his fear he may become assaultive and thus drive others away from him. He may do the reverse; he may withdraw from relations with others. Continuing fear might increase his suspiciousness of and inaccessibility to others. Finally, the patient's illness might become stabilized because his fear, in effect, reinforces his conception that others will make him uncomfortable, will hurt him; and he will become more convinced that he can derive no satisfaction from relating with other people.

« 2 »

Fear and Patient Assaultiveness

(continued)

WHY does a patient become assaultive? What can be done to reduce or eliminate this assaultiveness? How might it be handled when it does occur?

When a nurse is attacked by a patient she sometimes thinks that he is angry with her, dislikes her, or deliberately wants to hurt her. We have already suggested that though such an interpretation may be accurate in some instances, it is not necessarily always correct. There are other equally plausible interpretations. The patient may become assaultive because of an impulse he cannot control. He may be disoriented when he attacks, with no intention of hurting anyone in particular. The patient may mistake the nurse for someone else and attack her as if she were that person; thus, the attack is not personally directed at the nurse. We have already mentioned that the patient may become assaultive because he is frightened and attacks in the anticipation that others will hurt him. But we have not discussed a possibility that might impress the nurse as being strange, which is, that the patient's attack may be one of the few ways he has of having some contact with other people at that particular time. He may feel lonely and isolated and experience some need for physical contact and closeness with someone. He cannot express these needs verbally or in direct or conventional ways; he has to express them indirectly, hoping the nurse will recognize his needs and show concern for him. The patient may be afraid that he will not be taken care of, and he uses this desperate way of trying to get some of his needs satisfied. The patient may also attack the nurse when she neglects him, because she increases his loneliness and isolation. He may feel that she avoids him because she

44

believes him not to be worthwhile; this reinforces his feeling of worthlessness. It is understandable that he would attack someone who "makes" him feel unworthy.

It is in just these assaultive situations that the nurse finds it difficult to discover what his need is or give him the kind of relationship he may be seeking. Thus, it is important to recognize that the patient may be asking through his assaultiveness for some kind of experience or relation with the nurse that he is not getting. Once it is recognized that an attack is not necessarily *an attack on her* but could be *an appeal to her*, the nurse is better able to direct her attention to fulfilling the patient's needs in a way that is acceptable to him. It is through such fulfillment of needs that the nurse may help to reduce or eliminate the patient's assaultiveness.

HANDLING FEAR AND PATIENT ASSAULTIVENESS

Prevention of Patient Attack

A nurse may, by careful observation and appropriate action, prevent or interrupt a patient's assaultiveness. If she can discover for a particular patient the incidents or activities that lead up to assaultiveness, she might be able to anticipate it and help him overcome expressing himself in this way. Two illustrations follow:

> Mr. Adams sometimes became angry when he was denied a request and became assaultive if someone touched him. The nurses quickly learned not to touch Mr. Adams when he was angry and passed this information on to new members of the staff. If no one touched him, his anger usually subsided without a "blowup." The nurses also found that if they asked Mr. Adams to come to his room to talk, walked alongside him while returning to the room and sat with him for a little while, his anger would ordinarily disappear quite rapidly.

> When Mr. Bell was about to become assaultive, he usually indicated this by switching lights on and off, slamming doors, and taking on a "dark" look. Nurses recognized these signs and immediately asked him to talk with them in his room. Many times Mr. Bell's anger was interrupted by the nurse's coming to him, and he would quiet down quickly.

Nurses who have worked with a patient for some time are able to recognize signs of mounting tension and possible upset. Occasionally they can figure out ways of allaying his tension and preventing a physical assault. In the two examples given above, apparently the presence of a nurse and her willingness to talk with the patient were enough to interrupt an attack. Sometimes the solution is not that simple. The nurse may have to observe carefully the pattern of a patient's assaultiveness many times from its inception to the actual outbreak of the attack, before she can determine when and how she might interrupt the pattern.

There may be times when assaultiveness cannot be prevented, but the way in which any particular incident is handled is important. The way the nurse handles it may lay the foundation for future attacks (for example, if the nurse hits the patient back), or it may reduce the patient's need to be assaultive (for example, if she tells the patient she does not like to be hurt, if she talks to him, or if she stays with him in order to help reduce his fear or anxiety). Thus, the problem of reducing or eliminating patient assaultiveness has two aspects. One concerns dealing with a particular situation so that the potential or actual assault is handled adequately. The second concerns the kind of therapeutic relationship the nurse can form with the patient, both in the handling of his upset states and during other periods, that will make his attacks unnecessary.

The Nurses's Handling of Her Own Fear

We pointed out previously that a nurse who is afraid of a patient and communicates her fear to him may help to bring about his assaultiveness. The question we need to explore is: How can the nurse handle her own fear so that she is able to relate to the patient in a way that will not provoke his attack? Some illustrations may help to answer this question.

As a result of group and individual discussions, Miss Jones, an inexperienced nurse who had just come to the hospital, became curious about Mr. Jackson (a patient discussed in a previous illustration). She wondered what she might do to overcome her fear of him. She was especially troubled because his "excuse me" had such an ominous tone that it frightened her away. But after several group and individual discussions about her fear of this patient she gradually lost that fear. She was interviewed to find out what helped her overcome her fear of Mr. Jackson.

SOCIOLOGIST: How were you able to take Sam Jackson's "excuse me" without letting it bother you?

MISS JONES: We've been thinking of his "excuse me" as his meaning to dismiss us and threaten us. I don't believe that's it at all.

SOCIOLOGIST: It might mean something else?

MISS JONES: "Excuse me" may be an expression of a lot of things.

SOCIOLOGIST: What do you think changed in yourself that made you change your attitude toward him?

MISS JONES: I felt very strongly that if I searched my own behavior more thoroughly, I would discover something. I began to remember various reactions of his, and it was so interesting and beneficial!

SOCIOLOGIST: Can you tell me why and how it was interesting and beneficial?

MISS JONES: The fears I had of him disappeared. It was just amazing that first morning.

SOCIOLOGIST: You mean that morning when you just stood with him, then got him dressed, and he talked about the dog.

MISS JONES: I can't figure it out, but he just responded. I did a great deal of adjusting to the situation last Thursday (at the group meeting), and talking about it helped to clear me up some. I began really focusing on my relation to him, our relation together.

SOCIOLOGIST: What was it? Tell me more about what you learned that made your fear disappear.

MISS JONES: What Carol said came to my mind vividly. The way to get over fear of a patient is to spend more time with him, to find out what approach works with him and what approaches don't work. And if something doesn't work after several attempts, try something new. Before, if he said "excuse me" very loudly I would practically tremble. By spending more time with him I feel very comfortable. You heard him blasting [shouting] the other morning. I don't feel like running now when he does that. I wasn't expecting it, but I was able to say ,"All right, if you have to do that," or something like that. And the same thing happened today. Our relation hasn't been anything spectacular, but at least I haven't felt anxious about it. At one point he became very angry and spit in my face and told me to leave him alone. It frightened me for a minute, but I didn't run. I stood there and said, "Oh, Sam, I don't think you meant to do that really."

SOCIOLOGIST: You were really saying you didn't feel hurt by this.

MISS JONES: Yes, and I didn't feel like running. It's interesting for me to see this fear disappear. Also, I learned something about that.

SOCIOLOGIST: You learned something about what?

MISS JONES: About this feeling of fear you have with patients and how it's relayed to them. I think they can sense it very easily. After Sam spit at me I went out to get his shoes. When I came back he was pressing up against the door and wouldn't let me in. He came out shortly afterward and went on the porch. I felt good enough about it that I went out and told him I had found his shoes and said, "Come on, let's put them on." He said in a loud voice, "I don't want to have anything to do with you, please leave me alone." The first experience like that with him would have made me run. I would have been afraid he was going to hit me. But now I sat on the porch for a couple of minutes.

SOCIOLOGIST: You didn't leave?

MISS JONES: No. And then he laughed very loud and said, "Oh, I'll see you later." So I think he knows about all this fear that we have of him.

SOCIOLOGIST: He sure does.

MISS JONES: And whenever he knows you're not afraid and he can't chase you away, then he's willing to go along with you. I'm sure it makes him feel more comfortable when he knows that you're not afraid. And maybe it dispels some of his fear of having us so close to him.

SOCIOLOGIST: Can you be a little more specific about the step between the time you felt the fear and the time you lost it? What went on there?

MISS JONES: I think so. In the first place, I never had any relationship with him, none at all. If he would say, "Excuse me, please," I would excuse him. Then one morning I brought his tray and the dog (the ward pet) followed me in. I said good morning to him, and I wasn't planning to say anything else because I expected the usual reaction. And then he looked down at the dog and I saw he was interested in him. He started talking about the dog. And this interest he showed in the dog seemed to pave the way for me to ask him to come out on the porch and play with the dog. At the time I think my mind was focused on the fact that he was doing these things, not on my own fear. I think that I might have had a very slight awareness that the fear wasn't present at the time, but I think my mind was focused more on what he was doing. And the first time that I realized that I wasn't afraid and that I felt actually quite comfortable with him was later when we were out in the hall. There were a lot of people milling around, and I felt comfortable enough to put my arm around him and say, "Here we go." I mean it just seemed the thing to do, and I felt comfortable about it. And then later I thought, "Gee, I put my hand on his shoulder and I never even thought about it, and before I was so afraid of him." So I think that it was the things that he was doing, his responses, that made me feel less afraid, that he could accept my presence. That's what it seems to me went on.

SOCIOLOGIST: Well, it was a whole series of new experiences, then, that were quite different from those you had had previously or had anticipated. And you were able to take the experience because you were able to leave yourself open for it. If you had been put off by his "excuse me," you wouldn't have developed to this further stage. It's quite possible that on the next day, or another day, he wouldn't respond in the same way. But as long as you wait it's apt to come.

MISS JONES: I was quite aware of this. Miss Adams [a nurse] was saying, "You ought to receive a gold medal," and I said, "I don't think so, because it was really Sam who led me to feel this way or made it possible. So things just progressed.

SOCIOLOGIST: You shouldn't make that mistake either, that it's only Sam. It has to be the relationship between the two of you. It's neither you nor he, but it's both of you with each other.

MISS JONES: The other people on the ward also helped. I think that's important, too. Because I don't think it's Sam and me alone. I think it's a lot of things combined. It's been quite a learning experience for me.

SOCIOLOGIST: So many people are afraid to learn. Their anxiety is greater than their desire to learn. They would rather keep out of the situation and keep the anxiety down than get into it and create the possibility of its rising.

What seemed to help Miss Jones overcome her fear? She became curious about what she might be able to do with the patient and about the patient's way of keeping people away. Her curiosity led to seeing an alternative—that the patient's "excuse me" might mean something other than "keep away or I'll hit you." Then she became curious about herself—her own reactions to the patient and what the patient was doing to elicit these reactions. *She began to focus on their relationship—not on her fear of the patient.* She became interested in trying different approaches with the patient rather than concentrating on how fearful she was and on what she could do to avoid him. Her previous experiences with him and her expectations of him did not prevent her from having new and different experiences with the patient. When an opportunity arose to carry out a different relationship with the patient, she took advantage of it. Thus, she could spend more time with him, not be frightened off, and even be reassuring when necessary.

After Miss Jones went to another ward the sociologist talked with her about her experiences with assaultive patients on the new ward.

SOCIOLOGIST: I wonder if we could continue our talk about what was helpful to you in reducing your fear of patients.

MISS JONES: It's been diminished to a great extent through contacts with patients of whom I've been afraid and discussion in the group. You'll be interested to know that the discussion we had about fear helped me. Why are we really afraid? Do they hurt us seriously? What is this fear based on? Alice Evans [a patient] almost knocked my block off when I came on the ward yesterday. She hit me suddenly with both hands right in my face, very hard, but it didn't really hurt at all. I felt no pain. It surprised me at first and I didn't know what was going on, but I wasn't really afraid of her. I went over and stood by her until she calmed down and took my hand.

SOCIOLOGIST: That's very good. It proves the point, doesn't it, that if you're really not afraid and you show the patients you're not afraid, then they're not afraid of their own hostility and they can stop.

MISS JONES: The same thing happened with Shirley. I went into her room to get her to try on some brassieres. She was lying on the bed, so I stooped down and explained what I wanted and held out the brassieres. She took them and threw them back at me as hard as she could. So I picked them up and just stood there. She was really surprised—she had such an amazed expression on her face.

SOCIOLOGIST: Everybody runs when she does that.

MISS JONES: It was a definite look of amazement. I observed her very closely and she was really surprised.

SOCIOLOGIST: Did she say anything?

MISS JONES: Nothing. She grabbed the brassieres out of my hand and threw them at me again. But I just stayed there. Again she looked amazed. I didn't say anything, and neither did she. And then all of a sudden she burst into wild laughter. When she calmed down I asked her why she threw the brassieres at me—if she wanted to scare me. She looked at me very surprised. She didn't respond. It was the way she looked that mattered most. So I said, "I can see why you'd want to make me afraid, because *you* might be afraid." And I said, "I don't feel that way." I just stayed there for a long time, until I felt that that had passed over. Then I said, "Would you try on the brassieres for me now?" She said, "No." I said, "Maybe you will later?" She said, "Yes, I'll try them on later." I sat with her on the floor for about fifteen minutes and I thought it was quite a profitable experience on the whole.

SOCIOLOGIST: You must have felt very good about that, that you were able to handle yourself that way.

MISS JONES: I really did. I didn't get the brassieres tried on, but I felt I had accomplished more than that. I went in beaming all over to tell them about it in the office.

SOCIOLOGIST: It's good that you could let yourself lose sight of the immediate goal—that is, trying on the brassieres—for the more important one of establishing a relation with her where she knew you weren't afraid.

MISS JONES: That's something I've learned, too.

We have had reported to us many instances in which a nurse is *less* afraid of a patient *after* she has been attacked than she was *before.* It is important for nurses to recognize that their fear might be greater in anticipation than in the actual situation. In addition, a patient often *expects* the nurse to be afraid, and when she does not fulfill this expectation he may be both surprised and relieved and consequently have no need to attack her.

Recognizing the Patient's Desperation

In the following example a head nurse discusses her experiences with patients who are feared by many of the personnel.

SOCIOLOGIST: What's been going on with Joan these days? She seems to be attacking everyone.

HEAD NURSE: She's quite desperate. If she thinks nobody cares when she's desperate, she'll go to any length to find out if it's true, even to threats and assaults. She'll keep this up until it reaches a point where everyone is so hostile to her that the only sorts of feelings she gets from people are hostile ones. What happens? We end up by secluding her. When she has to act in such an aggressive way, it must mean our relationship with her is poor.

We had the same problem with Doris. We were told not to go near her when she became upset because she would hurt us. That didn't make any sense to me, so once I went to her when she was upset and said, "We aren't going to hurt you, and we won't let you hurt us." The other thing I told her that seemed to help was, "I'll stay with you until you feel better." She soon stopped shouting and thrashing around. I sat with her in her room, and she turned to me and said, "You know how sick I am." And she sat in the chair and held on to my arms. She said, "I'm terribly, terribly sick. Why don't you understand?" After this incident I've been able to handle three of her "blows" without secluding her.

SOCIOLOGIST: Do you realize what this means to personnel on the ward? This breaks down their attitude of fear when they see you do this and see what it does for the patient.

HEAD NURSE: After they see something like this they come and ask what happened and express interest in what I did.

SOCIOLOGIST: Are they any less frightened?

HEAD NURSE: No, they haven't overcome their fear, but they're at least able to observe that something different goes on. I brought out that I wondered if the reason I didn't get hit is that I felt she wouldn't hit me.

SOCIOLOGIST: The other side of this is that the patient here is actually terribly frightened of what he's going to do to the other person, and so when personnel are frightened or show fear, they reinforce the patient's idea that he will be murderous. Part of our obligation is to protect the patient from his own feelings, and you can't do that by having those fearful attitudes.

HEAD NURSE: If we can stay with Doris and make it possible for her to handle her feelings, this helps her with her opinion of herself. If every time she does this we lock her up, it makes her feel that she's a pretty despicable, dangerous character and has no ability to control herself.

SOCIOLOGIST: I'm interested in what you do with the personnel after an incident like this one with Doris.

HEAD NURSE: They come into the office and say, "What's wrong with her that she has to hit everybody?"

SOCIOLOGIST: But they do come into the office and ask you about it, and do you make yourself available right afterward?

HEAD NURSE: Yes, I try to.

SOCIOLOGIST: That's a good idea.

HEAD NURSE: All you need is one person who isn't afraid, to lead the others, and if you don't have one on a disturbed ward, your ward just goes to pot.

We frequently find that a circular process is maintained by the nurse and patient which continues the patient's assaultiveness. It goes like this: The patient is assaultive. The nurse does not recognize or experience the patient's desperation; she feels only his hostility. The nurse responds with hostility to the patient and may punish him in some way. This action reinforces the patient's need to keep on being assaultive, which in turn reinforces the nurse's need to be restrictive and punishing. Thus, a circular pattern is established in which both are hostile toward each other and neither is changing his or her behavior.

It is inevitable that at times the nurse will become angry with patients. She cannot exercise control over *what* she feels, although she might be able to control the *expression of her feelings*. We believe that it is possible for the nurse to develop an understanding of her feelings and impulses and thereby handle them in such a way that hostile activity toward the patient will be unnecessary. We have found that important changes may occur when a nurse is given an opportunity to talk openly about her feelings without fear of being blamed or punished, and in a spirit of trying to find a way to handle her feelings most usefully for herself and the patient. As a result of such discussion, she may find out what her feelings are based on and perhaps discover that she has mixed feelings toward the patient. She may become curious about her feelings, asking herself and finding out how they work, what they are related to, and how they might be changed. She might eventually find that the intensity of her feelings is reduced. As a matter of fact, her angry, hostile feelings may be so diminished that she may be able to approach the patient with many more ideas about how she might be helpful to him.

Situations of continuing hostility between a patient and various staff members can be interrupted if only one nurse reacts differently. The interruption of this pattern may be especially effective if this nurse is in a position of authority. If one nurse reacts toward the patient who is assaultive not with hostility but with some understanding of his desperate state and his great need for reassurance, she may be able to break up the pattern of conflict and thereby help the patient reduce or eliminate his need to be assaultive. This nurse may also serve as an example for other personnel. Through discussion and explanation of why the patient's assaultiveness continues and why it stops when the nurse takes a different attitude and approach toward him, other personnel may learn how to deal differently with him.

Irrational Patient Attacks

We indicated previously that sometimes a patient attacks a nurse because he mistakes her for someone else. If the nurse realizes that the attack may not be directed at her personally, she may be a little more accepting of the patient. In the example below a nurse tells how she handled Miss Carroll after this patient attacked her.

> MISS CROFT: I went back to her room to see what was going on, and she [Miss Carroll] said to me, "This isn't my blouse." I said, "It's the blouse that your mother sent you a month or so ago—it's yours." She said, "I don't want anything that my mother has to send to me." She grabbed me by the neck and started choking. I got her hands off my neck and held her arms, but she got hold of my watch and pulled it off and hit me a few times. Then she quieted down and went over and sat down on the mattress. That all happened yesterday. So today I was in with her and I brought it up. I said, "Do you remember what happened yesterday?" She said, "Yes." I said, "Was that directed at me personally?" She said, "Oh, no," and then started rambling on about something else. I had the impression that she hallucinated me to be her mother, or something. I didn't know for sure.
>
> SOCIOLOGIST: It would seem to me from the way you describe this situation that she was getting you mixed up with somebody else— that you happened to be there, that's all. The thing that surprised me a little bit was that she recalled it.
>
> MISS CROFT: I expected that when I asked her about it she would pass it off as she does so many questions that you ask her and just ramble on about something else. But she did give me a direct answer. She did say that she remembered it. And when I asked her if it was directed at me personally, she did say no.
>
> SOCIOLOGIST: The interesting thing there from the point of view of nursing is the feeling that you had. It was very important for you to go back and see her because you didn't want to become afraid.
>
> MISS CROFT: Yes, I didn't want to become afraid of her. I wanted to go back in with her.
>
> SOCIOLOGIST: I wonder if that point is impressed enough on the personnel—that after they are attacked, if they can possibly bring themselves to see the patient soon afterward and maybe get some things straightened out, they won't have to keep away from the patient.
>
> MISS CROFT: I wanted to go back yesterday, but things happened so that I couldn't make it. I was leery of going in today, you know,

because I didn't know whether the attack was directed at me or not, and so I left the door open.

SOCIOLOGIST: You felt sort of apprehensive, but on the other hand you wanted to do it.

A nurse can often straighten out her relationship with a patient after an attack by discussing it with him. If he is reluctant to talk about the situation, she need not push it but at least can indicate her interest in talking it over. Coming to the patient may help him feel that he has not driven her away or that his attack was not so horrible that it could not even be discussed.

Sometimes a nurse becomes distressed when a patient is assaultive because she thinks his assaultiveness is her fault and that she should have been able to prevent it. However, at times patients are assaultive despite our best efforts. At such times the patient may be reacting to voices and fantasies that tell him to attack the other person. Neither the patient nor the nurse can control these voices and prevent the attack. However, *the occurrence of an attack may not be so important as the way it is handled*. If the nurse can reduce her concern over the fact that the patient was assaultive, she might be able to focus on the important interpersonal relationship she is having with the patient in the situation. This relationship contributes to their future relationships, and what is done and felt in it may influence the patient's need to continue his assaultiveness. On the one hand, the nurse may handle the attack with the attitude that she does not like to get hit, but in rejecting the behavior she is not rejecting the patient. She is so interested in the patient that she wants to find out what makes it necessary for him to continue being assaultive and what she can do to change these assault-producing circumstances. On the other hand, she can reject the patient, remain frightened of him, and treat him as though he were some kind of terrible creature. The former way of dealing with the patient is more likely than the latter to reduce the patient's assaultiveness. We mean, of course, not that the assaultiveness is reduced because the patient is punished or forcibly made to stop his behavior, but that the patient gives it up because the nurse's relationship with him makes its continuation unnecessary.

Reacting Conventionally to an Attack

We pointed out previously that one of the major problems personnel have in dealing with patients stems from the cultural patterns they bring with them into the hospital. Some of the ways of acting that are acceptable and necessary in ordinary living simply do not apply if a nurse is to deal with a patient therapeutically.

In the following illustration the sociologist and a supervisor are discussing some problems in getting personnel to see that some of the reactions and approaches they use in ordinary life may not be applicable in their dealings with patients.

> SOCIOLOGIST: Outside, if someone screams at you and attacks you, what do you do? Either you scream and shout back at him, or you hit him back, or you ignore him, or you feel hurt. But what you're supposed to do when a patient does it in a mental hospital is to accept it, not get personally involved, not take it to heart, try to understand what is behind it, and react in a way completely different from the way you would react if you were on the outside. Now this is a terrifically difficult transition, it would seem to me, for the personnel to make. They live in this outside world; they're part of it; they've already built up these attitudes and reactions to a situation like this, and yet they come and work in a mental hospital and they're expected to do something completely different.
>
> SUPERVISOR: We expect them to understand and to accept and to go along with some patients.
>
> SOCIOLOGIST: They have to be flexible; they have to adjust and readjust all the time, and they have to be able to take the demands made on them.
>
> SUPERVISOR: The question is: How *do* you work with personnel so that they can accomplish what we want?
>
> SOCIOLOGIST: You can do it through training, through seeing it work on the ward, and through discussion around specific incidents as they arise. You have to surround the personnel the same way that you surround the patient. The patient is surrounded by a certain set of attitudes, and we want to surround him with a different set. We want personnel to change their attitudes; we want them to develop attitudes that are much more acceptable to psychiatric patients.

The significant point of this illustration is that personnel in the mental hospital must recognize that they have to participate somewhat differently with mental patients from the way they do with people outside the hospital. Nurses have to carry on a continuous adjustment and readjustment in many of their attitudes toward, feelings about, and approaches to patients if they are to be of maximum use to them.

Group Support

Of great importance in helping the nurse handle a patient's assaultiveness adequately is the assistance she gets from her co-workers. If their support is forthcoming at the right time and in an appropriate way, the nurse may be more secure in dealing with the patient.

SOCIOLOGIST: What can we do about that matter of feeling all alone when you're struggling with a combative patient?

MISS ADAMS: One thing that helps me is knowing the holds on how best to handle these patients.

MISS BELL: Even if you're not too sure of the best hold, if others get in there and help—grab her leg if she's kicking—it lessens the over-all fear. The patient feels more secure and you feel more secure, and you won't have this feeling, "Well, nobody bothers about what's going to happen to me."

MRS. ALLEN: It's that horrible feeling the first two or three minutes when a patient attacks you. It seems like two or three years before somebody gets there to help you.

SOCIOLOGIST: It's the immediacy of the help that's important— someone coming right at the very moment when you need it most. Of course, you wish you could prevent the attack from happening altogether.

MISS ADAMS: You can't prevent some things from happening. I don't think any particular attack is terribly important. I think the way it is handled is much more important than the fact of the attack. But I think you feel better about it if you know at least that your fellow workers are rallying around and trying to help instead of going into another room.

MRS. ALLEN: I'm scared when anything like that happens.

MISS BELL: I'm scared afterward.

SOCIOLOGIST: If you really learn to work together, and after you've handled a couple of difficult situations together and you've done it effectively, you are confident that you can do it. If you've never actually had a team working in these situations, then you don't know what it's like.

In these assaultive situations the nurse's security is usually threatened. One way in which she can maintain her security, as well as develop it, is to have the experience of giving and getting support from others in difficult situations. Assaults by patients create dependence of one nurse upon another, and a nurse needs the confidence derived from the assurance that others will pitch in and do their share.

Reducing a Patient's Assaults

In our previous discussion of the ways a patient's assaultiveness might be handled we did not sufficiently emphasize the importance of getting to know the patient by dealing with him over a period of time. When the nurse becomes familiar with the patient's ways, when she knows some of the circumstances that provoke his assaultiveness and some of the things that calm him when he is upset, she may develop security and skill in coping with these situations. Not only is her knowledge and familiarity with a particular patient useful, but her experience with many assaultive patients in a variety of situations will help her acquire skill and confidence in handling them effectively.

In order to illustrate personnel experiences with an assaultive patient over a period of time we present a series of examples dealing with Mrs. Board. This patient's assaultiveness aroused great fear among personnel and considerable conference time was spent discussing her. In these examples, the feelings of both the patient and the nurses will be shown, and the various attempts to deal with Mrs. Board's assaultiveness will be described. Participating in the first conference are the sociologist, three nurses, two aides, and four student nurses.

October 2

SOCIOLOGIST: Do you think it would be of some value to try to talk about what could be done to handle Mrs. Board's aggressiveness, or what could be done to make it unnecessary?

MISS ALLEN: I'd like to hear from some of the students.

MISS ABEL: We talk about her in class all the time.

MISS ALLEN: Before you came to the ward, how did you feel about her? Had she been discussed in class?

Miss Abel: We got the idea there that she's likely to attack us.

Miss Allen: And how did you feel about that?

Miss Best: We were a little worried and didn't want to be around her.

Miss Carr: Before I came to the ward I was scared to death of her.

Sociologist: Because of what you heard?

Miss Carr: Because of what I heard and what I've seen, too. I saw the marks on other students.

Sociologist: How about you, Miss Dunn?

Miss Dunn: I'm sort of afraid to be too close to her, but I like her. I don't know why.

Miss Allen: I was wondering if you had any suggestions as to what we might do.

Miss Broome: We were talking about the possibilities, and some of the people thought we ought to tell her off when she did anything to us.

Sociologist: Tell her off? How?

Miss Broome: Instead of fighting her with your fists, fight her with words.

Mrs. Ames: I disagree. I think when she's in that mood that she wouldn't pay any attention to what you say.

Miss Broome: The other day when I talked rather mean to her she really looked frightened.

Miss Cress: If we were as frightened as she is, we'd probably strike back first.

Sociologist: If it's fear on her part, then what would be the best way to handle her fear, if that's what we're dealing with instead of aggressiveness?

Miss Broome: I don't think it's really aggressiveness, do you?

Miss Allen: Well that's the way it comes out when she throws her tray, but I don't think it's because she really wants to hurt anybody.

Mrs. Brenner: She doesn't like to think that you know she's afraid.

Mrs. Ames: She told me one day that we were all out to kill her and that she was going to kill us first. So it's pretty clear how afraid she is.

Miss Allen: If we could figure out a way to get her over feeling like this, we'd also solve how we could get over feeling she may fly at us every time we turn our backs.

Sociologist: What can we do to get her over her feelings and us over our own feelings?

Miss Allen: When really disturbed children become aggressive, the one thing that works very well is some statement to the effect that you aren't going to let them be hurt and you aren't going to let them hurt you.

MISS BROOME: That is also effective with combative patients. I've used it.

SOCIOLOGIST: It strikes me that since she often throws her tray in the morning, wouldn't it be wise the first time you go in to ask, "Is it all right to come in now?" I wonder how many of the patients feel that you barge in on them and they don't have any privacy at all.

MISS ALLEN: I think you should knock on a patient's door.

SOCIOLOGIST: After you knock you might ask to come in. This indicates you're showing a patient some respect, and if she is in a bad mood you'll know it right away.

MRS. AMES: Suppose she says, "No."

SOCIOLOGIST: Then you can say, "What's up? Why not?"

MRS. BRENNER: Maybe you could say, "Ready for breakfast?"

SOCIOLOGIST: If anybody has any more ideas I'd like to hear them.

MISS ALLEN: I would think after she throws her tray or does something aggressive, somebody ought to go in immediately and try to find out what's troubling her or why she's frightened.

MISS BROOME: I've done that and she tells me, "I don't want to talk about it," or, "It's not your fault, don't feel so bad about it, don't feel so responsible," or else, "My mind is exposed. You can read my mind. You're trying to kill me and I'm going to kill you first." These are three different answers that she's given me, but never anything specific about the incident.

SOCIOLOGIST: Well, I wouldn't worry about the answer. I think just the fact that you do it is important to her, even though she may not tell you. She probably doesn't know why herself, but at least she knows you're interested enough to come in. The worst thing about hitting somebody is that you feel so terrible about it yourself. "Oh, how could I have been so mean to this other person." But if this other person then comes back to you and says, "Well, it wasn't so terrible," then your own guilt subsides and you don't feel so bad about it. I think the same thing goes on with her. If you come back and say, "I'm really interested in finding out what's wrong," then I think she can feel a little better about it, and this may help in the long run. I wouldn't expect too much of an answer.

The discussion of the patient continues, this time by a doctor, two nurses, and the sociologist.

October 11

DR. ASHTON: I hear Mrs. Board continues to be assaultive, that she's been hitting people. She's very much isolated, staying in her room.

SOCIOLOGIST: When personnel go into her room she pops up and hits them. She tore the uniform off Evans [an aide] on Saturday, and people are now getting so terrified they don't want to go near her.

MISS ALLEN: You just mention her name, and they don't want to have anything to do with her.

MISS BROOME: So we restricted her privileges after she hit Evans the second time.

SOCIOLOGIST: I think here's a way the patient gets herself surrounded with fear, and she's bound to lose. I just wonder if we can come up with any bright ideas as to what to do with her.

MISS BROOME: She's been noticing how we've taken care of some of the other patients, and that makes her angry. She attacked Mrs. Black [a patient] when we were paying her a lot of attention. The other day she remarked to one of the new nurses, "It seems like all the patients' needs are taken care of but mine. Nobody even has any idea of what mine are." She said this to a gal who is brand new on the ward and with whom she's had very little contact, and then ordered her out of the room.

MISS ALLEN: She's been more aggressive verbally to me lately. The other morning I smiled at her and she said, "Don't smile at me like a hyena." It's got to the point where you don't know what to do. She's terrified, she's anxious. You have a feeling you'd like to go up and say, "Well now look here, we're going to take care of you and do something about this; you're not going to go on like this." You have a feeling this is what she wants you to do, but you feel there's a circle drawn around her and you'd better not step inside that circle. I've got so now I'm just scared to even smile out of one corner of my mouth at her.

SOCIOLOGIST: I would like to see if we could get a consistent program with her. When you go in there and she orders you out and you feel she's pretty much terrified, I wonder if it wouldn't be a good idea to stay in there and say, "I'm going to stay with you because I feel you can use some company," or "you can use somebody around,"— and do this consistently over a long period of time.

MISS ALLEN: It all depends on how she tells me to get out, whether I do or not. There are lots of times when she tells me to leave and I don't, but there are other times when she tells me to leave and I do.

SOCIOLOGIST: I think she told us quite directly that she really wants people to stay with her when she said, "You know how to take care of everybody else but me." She might need this more elementary care. Another thing is that she can be warm and friendly. I think the tendency is to discount that and concentrate on the idea that she's a horrible person who is beating everybody up.

DR. ASHTON: Does she continue an attack after she starts it, or is it just one sock, and then she stops?

MISS ALLEN: If nobody comes she'll continue. She battered a student up one day—bruised her cheek and scratched her.

SOCIOLOGIST: If we work on the idea that the patient is more terrified than you are, that she is really very frightened and wants somebody to comfort her, then our problem is: How do we get things organized so that personnel don't get mutilated and at the same time the patient feels somebody understands her and is attending to her needs.

MISS ALLEN: We might even tell her that we can't have people hurt any longer, that we recognize that she has an impulse to hurt people. This might be something the doctor and the head nurse could handle in a joint conference with her. Then two of us would go in and we'd try to carry out this idea that we weren't going to let her hurt anyone, although we recognized her feelings.

MISS BROOME: I think we ought to present this idea to the rest of the ward staff.

In an interview with the sociologist a head nurse tells of her attempts to get an aide to try to understand some of his reactions to Mrs. Board. The aide is young, new on the ward, and trying to figure out his relations with patients.

October 16

HEAD NURSE: When Jack Cooper [the aide] took Mrs. Board downstairs she called him no end of names and shouted, "Don't stand near me!" On the elevator she spit at him and he told her nobody ever spit on him and got by with it. She called him some more names, and by the time they got downstairs they were screaming at each other. Dr. Hillman [who saw the incident] told me that Jack was about to haul off and hit her, he was so mad. He was just furious when he came back upstairs. He started this tirade—nobody was going to spit on him and get by with it! When she got back to the floor he was really going to give it to her. I listened to all this and then I asked him if he thought that hitting her would help. He said he could hit her without hurting her. He said, "If you let patients know you would hit them, then you can deal with them after that. You might as well let them know, it's only fair to them. Let them know where they stand and this will teach them quicker than anything else." So I just let him go on, and then he asked me if I had ever hit a patient. I said, "No." He said that was the trouble with me, I was too good to the patients. I then pointed out where I had set limits for patients—what I thought were reasonable limits, and he agreed to that. I spent a lot of time with him that night. I tried to get him to see what had happened to the schizophrenic and what we were up against with many patients who were paranoid—what their solution in life had become, and how this sort of thing would reinforce it.

SOCIOLOGIST: How did he react?

HEAD NURSE: He didn't agree with me, but he had some idea of what I was getting at. But then Dr. Hillman came upstairs and explained her behavior to me, him, and Lawrence [another aide]. He said Mrs. Board's spitting and hitting is an automatic reaction. She believes everybody is against her and hates her, and the reason she does this is that her mother constantly spit at her. Then he explained to Jack that she probably had some friendly feelings toward him, but she couldn't accept them because they made her too anxious. She had to do something about it and tell him off to get rid of those feelings. Then Dr. Hillman said that the people on the ward stand for people that she's had experiences with in the past, that it isn't a personal thing. He was trying to get Jack to see that. Dr. Hillman said, "When she spit at you there was nothing personal about it; that is her reaction to all people she feels friendly toward." He suggested we treat her in a matter-of-fact way. Afterward I had a short talk with Jack. He said, "It certainly makes a lot of difference in how I feel. I certainly didn't understand this before. I feel very different about it now." Later on in the day before he went home he said he wanted to talk to me. He said, "Forget what I said about hitting her. It wouldn't work. I've just been thinking about it, and it wouldn't work."

A few days later the nurse reports another conversation with the aide.

October 19

HEAD NURSE: The other night Lenore [a patient] blew up and was raging in a loud voice at him [the aide]. She hit him in the face and it was all red blotches. He came in to talk about it with me later. He said she began swearing and screaming at him and then hit him. He got furious, but didn't do anything. He finally came out and said he wasn't really afraid of the patient, but he got so angry that he was afraid of what he would do to her. Then he reassured me that he had hit a patient only once, and he had a lot of guilt about it and wished he had had someone to talk to then. I told him that being afraid of our own anger was true for many of us and that it took a lot of experience and talking about how one really felt. I also said I noticed that he seemed to get most angry not when a patient did something to him physically but when she made some disparaging remark about him. He said this was true. So we talked again about taking things personally and that he had to remember that patients were reacting to experiences that they had had in the past—that it wasn't really a reflection of what the nurse or aide had done, usually, but something that had been building up for a long time. Flaring back at them only reinforced it. His feeling about Mrs. Board came up again. He said he thought now that if she spit at him he could understand it.

Before his talk with the nurse Jack felt angry and resentful toward Mrs. Board. He experienced her attack as a blow to his self-esteem. In addition, he was concerned about what he might do to the patient because of his anger. He also felt guilty about his hostile feelings toward her. During their conferences the head nurse recognized his guilt and did not condemn him when he expressed his feelings. Rather, she listened and tried to throw some light on the patient's feelings and attitudes. During the discussions Jack was able to get a different perspective on "what the patient was up to," as well as to see his own concern about being disparaged by the patient. After the conferences Jack saw the patient's assaultiveness in a different way. He felt better about her and no longer responded with the feeling that he was being personally insulted by Mrs. Board's attacks.

Although Jack felt better about Mrs. Board's assaultiveness, many of the personnel persisted in their fear and avoidance of her, and the patient continued her attacks.

October 28

Miss Allen: We have noticed that Mrs. Board doesn't "jump" anyone when there are two people present, that it's always when one person is there alone.

Mrs. Ames: Well it seems to me that Mrs. Board gets very uneasy when there's somebody with her, or close to her. And if there are two people around, it doesn't seem to bother her as it does when there's one.

Miss Allen: I think she can tolerate two much more easily than one.

Miss Broome: She has come right out and said that we seem to be very interested in all the other patients' needs and what they want, and we know what to do to take care of them, but nobody seems to know what she needs. So there is a feeling on her part that we don't take care of her.

Mrs. BLAIR: I think we've seen that she is jealous of other patients. She has tried to interfere when another patient has been really sick and demanded a lot of care.

Miss ALLEN: We take care of all the other patients, but we've never got around to doing it with her. She's stuck and we're stuck.

Dr. ASHTON: I have the feeling that among all of us there's a certain amount of resentment against Mrs. Board. I've had it at times. I don't have it particularly at present, but I never have much contact with her.

Mrs. AMES: I used to have a lot of resentment toward her, more so than I do now. I still resent her spitting on the floor, but she hasn't gotten under my skin as she did last spring.

Miss ALLEN: There's a lot of feeling about her.

Dr. ASHTON: How do you feel about her, Mrs. Blair?

Mrs. BLAIR: There was a time that I didn't care to even be anywhere near her, but I don't mind her any more.

Mr. COOPER: Well, I used to stay away from her because I was afraid if I'd go anywhere near her I was going to end up hitting her.

Miss BROOME: I have stayed just as far away from her as I could. I got tired of having trays thrown at me and being attacked twice a day.

Mrs. BLAIR: It just puts tension on the whole ward when she's out of her room.

Miss ALLEN: It's a tradition that's been built around her, for one thing—that she's so dangerous, and yet actually she's just a little peewee, who can't be as dangerous as the picture is painted. I think it's our feelings of what we might do to her.

SOCIOLOGIST: Miss Sims, tell us how you feel.

Miss SIMS: I like her. I've wanted to put my arms around her and comfort her.

Mrs. DRAKE: I'd rather put my arms around a black snake.

Mr. COOPER: You don't know exactly what her reaction is going to be. She's so unpredictable.

Miss ALLEN: But she has a very warm, friendly side to her nature which comes out now and then.

Dr. ASHTON: I wonder what happened, Mrs. Drake, that you've come to feel that she's like a black snake and you wouldn't want to put your arms around her.

Mrs. DRAKE: After she threw about three or four trays at me, I just stayed away from her. I'm scared of her.

DR. ASHTON: Scared you will hit her with something?

MRS. DRAKE: I guess that's it, too, but I'm scared of her.

MISS ALLEN: I think what's probably behind so many of our feelings is that we're going to retaliate. Not that we're so afraid of her physically, but afraid of our feelings about her.

At one point during the period under discussion a number of patients in addition to Mrs. Board were assaultive. The head nurse and the sociologist discuss the upset ward situation, wondering what has brought about this rather widespread combativeness.

November 1

SOCIOLOGIST: What's going on with the patients and what are we doing with them to bring on this aggressive behavior? One of the things I've noticed is that the person who gets hit most of the time is Mrs. Drake, and she's the one who's most afraid. Also a lot of the students are getting hit.

HEAD NURSE: Maybe it's because they come to the ward frightened.

SOCIOLOGIST: But what does a ward do to get into a situation where aggression becomes a problem—especially when ordinarily it's no great problem—at least not a consistent problem?

HEAD NURSE: Well one thing is that aggression is not handled immediately and not handled directly. I don't mean that you would do anything to the patients as a means of restraining them, but rather when a patient is becoming upset, say, "Well you go to your room now, and I'll be with you." Something like this happened with Mrs. Rand [an aide] the other day. Mary [a patient] got upset, became loud, and hit Mr. Wilkins [another patient]. Mrs. Rand went into her room with her immediately and sat down with her, and Mary quieted down. I think this is what we ought to do with Mrs. Board and Sally—go immediately to them when they get upset.

SOCIOLOGIST: Every time after Mrs. Board blows up she gets friendly. Maybe it's because she feels guilty about it and wants the other person to show her it wasn't so horrible. But it might also mean that the only time you can notice she gets friendly is when you have contact with her. The question is how you can help people overcome their fear of that sort of violence, so that they can go in and withstand the danger, whatever it might be.

HEAD NURSE: When the feeling you get on the ward is that nobody will help you, that makes you more frightened.

SOCIOLOGIST: Because you can't rely on the other personnel.

HEAD NURSE: It's important to know that the other person is right with you when the patient gets upset.

SOCIOLOGIST: With Mrs. Board, people don't rush in to help, they just stand around watching or they try to get away from the situation.

HEAD NURSE: When they hear something going on they run into the office. The other day when Mrs. Board got out of her room, everybody went to the back or into the office.

SOCIOLOGIST: You can see how terrified they are of her. They're afraid to go into the living room when she's there.

HEAD NURSE: I think one of the main things is that fear calls out aggressive behavior. When I was at another hospital, the only time we really had any difficulty with our disturbed ward was when we had a supervisor who was scared of her shadow, and she communicated this to everyone else.

SOCIOLOGIST: This fear only increases the patient's necessity for doing something aggressive. People run away, and the running indicates how really frightened they are. This means to the patient that he can't get his needs fulfilled.

HEAD NURSE: It's an interesting cycle. Mrs. Board frightens the staff because of her own aggressive behavior. Then it's easy for her to project and say, "They're all inhuman, trying to grind me down and beat me around." When you point out to her that she's the one that's being aggressive she says, "No, they are." She objects to a student breathing near her and then hits the student for being nasty and breathing on her. She puts all the aggression on the personnel and you get a circle you can't break out of.

After the general ward upset subsided, some of the personnel became less fearful of Mrs. Board. At a ward staff conference the sociologist tried to explain to other personnel the way the patient appeared to him.

November 8

SOCIOLOGIST: I wonder if it would be helpful if I told you something I found out today about Mrs. Board, which I hadn't been able to put together before and which helped me understand her better. She keeps talking about everybody being murderous here and that she is being ground down and persecuted and what have you. You know whenever you ask her, "Well, what specifically is being done to you?" she'll come out with something about "they" make her work so hard. There are all these vague things that I couldn't quite make out. Now today she came out with something that helped me understand what she's talking about. She said, "The parents of the patients here look upon them [and she is talking about herself, I imagine, primarily] as being useless, they no longer want them, they want to get rid of them. So they put them in a mental hospital and they let them stay indefinitely, so that the doctors become the agents of the parents to get rid of these people [the patients] on the parents' instigation." That's why the patients are here, and that's why she feels the personnel, the doctors, and the nurses are all out to eliminate her. This is what she told me today; I had never heard her say it before or put it together this way. No matter what you do, you're a murderer.

MISS BROOME: As far as dealing with her, the only thing that helped me in the least to keep from slugging her or getting really mad at her was the conference last week at which I expressed my feelings, and I think pretty generally the feelings on the ward, that we just frustrate her and we are damned if we do and we're damned if we don't. Regardless of how we deal with her, it's the wrong way. It can't ever possibly be the right way. It was pointed out in the conference that all we can do is to offer her what we have—to do our best. That's all we can do.

In the final discussion that we present, some personnel are still afraid of Mrs. Board; others now have changed their attitudes and feelings.

November 15

SOCIOLOGIST: The way Mrs. Board's mind works, at least some part of the time, is that everybody is plotting against her, and a few weeks ago she told me the chief plotter was Mrs. Drake [an aide]. I think that she feels Mrs. Drake's fear more than anybody else's, because Mrs. Drake is really afraid to go in there to see her. Anyhow she feels that every minute of the day, even when we're at home, we are all planning ways and means of breaking her down, ruining her intelligence, making her crazy. When I say to her "Look, our purpose is to make you uncrazy," she sometimes doesn't hear that. When I asked her today, "Is this happening all the time?" she said, "No, most of the time though." When I asked her, "When doesn't it happen?" then she backtracked and said, "Well, it happens all the time." Then when I asked her, "Does it happen with everybody?" she says, "No, it doesn't happen with everybody. There are some people that it doesn't happen with." So I think it's rather interesting to get the picture from her angle. This is how she feels about the people around her. At one point I asked her, "Well, why would these people want to break you down the way you say they are trying to do?" She said that she knew lots of different reasons. Among them was the one I mentioned last week, that after all the parents are paying the bills. We are being employed by the hospital, which is being employed by the parents, in the sense that they are paying the bills. Therefore, we are employees of the parents and so are doing the parents' bidding. She said that her mother is such a hateful creature, that she wants to ruin her daughter. Well, this is Mrs. Board's attitude toward the world, and that's why she is in a mental hospital. This is her feeling about what goes on, and, she has evidence for it when we seclude her or restrain her from beating anybody up. When I tried to point out to her that she doesn't get restrained until she has done something against the personnel, she couldn't see it that way. I told her that she has all this stuff in her mind and as soon as people approach her, she does the same thing to them that she thinks that they are doing to her. I can't tell how much this penetrates. Sometimes I feel that it does. Sometimes I think that just for a moment this means something to her, and then it's lost.

I think some of my experiences with her might help us figure out what we can do to prevent her from getting into these assaultive wrangles with the staff. Anyway it's worth talking about our attitudes toward her. A lot of you feel that Mrs. Board is a very hostile, very frightening kind of person. I think it's interesting to get a different point of view, because I don't feel as you do at all. I think part of the problem all of us get stuck in is that we see the patient only from one angle. So those of you who feel that she is pretty hostile see that, and find it difficult to see her gentleness or warmth. Although I see Mrs. Board attack people, I also see that she is a very warm person, very friendly, very bright, and a lot of fun. Do you see or feel there is any warm, tender side to her at all, or is that impossible for you to see?

MRS. AMES: Well I try to see, but it's hard.

SOCIOLOGIST: It is rather hard. Have you had any experiences with her that have been at all successful?

MRS. AMES: Yes.

SOCIOLOGIST: What kind of experiences were they? Can you remember specifically the type of situation, what you were doing, what she was doing?

MISS BROOME: I remember one, when I gave her a permanent, which took a whole afternoon, and she sat very quietly in a big group and had a wonderful time.

SOCIOLOGIST: How about you, Mrs. Blair?

MRS. BLAIR: I'm to the point now where I can go in and sit with her and she will tell me that she'll never get well and that she's hopeless.

MRS. DRAKE: I don't want to go near her.

SOCIOLOGIST: Why?

MRS. DRAKE: I'm not comfortable.

SOCIOLOGIST: It seems to be a circular pattern. If you are uncomfortable when you do go near her she picks that up right away and makes you more uncomfortable, and so on. So the problem is how do you get less uncomfortable?

MRS. DRAKE: Stay away from her.

MISS BROOME: Yeah, but that wouldn't be very helpful.

SOCIOLOGIST: I wonder if you also see how terribly frightened she is. Sometimes I go in there and she is really trembling, and she'll say, "Stay near me," and she'll just huddle up close to me and say, "I'm terribly afraid."

Conferences and discussions about Mrs. Board continued, with a gradual lessening of fear among the personnel. Approximately six months after these discussions began, this patient left the disturbed ward; personnel were no longer afraid of her and she no longer assaulted them.

In our discussion thus far we have focused on a number of questions concerning fear and patient assaultiveness: What contributes to the nurse's fear? What contributes to the patient's fear? What contributes to the initiation and continuation of patient assaultiveness? How are fear and assaultiveness related? What can the nurse do to prevent, reduce, or eliminate the patient's fear and assaultiveness? Although we have dealt with this problem situation at considerable length, we do not mean to imply that "Fear and Patient Assaultiveness" is necessarily the most important type of problem situation that arises in the mental hospital. We have put it first and we have dealt with it extensively so that it might be used as a model for examining and analyzing other types of problem situations that we do not explore so fully.

Once a patient becomes assaultive, a circular process may be established in which the nurse becomes afraid; her fear stimulates the patient's fear and his further assaultiveness; the assaultiveness reinforces the nurse's fear; and this fear elicits further attacks from the patient. In this circular situation, assaultiveness remains a central problem. The reason we call this a problem situation may now be clearer. Both patient and nurse contribute to the situation by the way they deal with each other. The situation is maintained because these reciprocal patterns of activity continue with little variation or interruption.

Since the nurse's fear contributes conspicuously to the continuation of these stable situations, we have focused on how she acquires and maintains her fear and on what can be done to reduce it. We have found it helpful for the nurse to develop a questioning attitude toward her feelings and toward the relations between herself and the patient. If she can look at the kinds of activities that contribute to patient aggressiveness and the kinds of situations that make it unnecessary for patients to be assaultive, she may learn how the circular pattern gets established. Such a recognition may help her reduce her fear of the patient, interrupt the circular pattern, and thus reduce or eliminate the assaultive behavior.

If the nurse can examine the situations of patient assaultiveness from the various perspectives we have indicated, she may find it easier to resolve these situations to her own and the patient's benefit. We would like the nurse to look upon our suggestions as possible alternatives in these situations and to determine for herself how much of her experience corresponds to ours and the extent to which the ideas and approach presented here are applicable to her own nursing situation.

« 3 »

The Patient Is Demanding

PERIODICALLY, a particular patient or several patients become the focus of attention because of their insistent requests. As these requests continue, the nurse may come to feel that they are more than she can reasonably meet, and she may label the patient "a demanding patient." If other personnel also share this view of a patient, he may acquire a reputation of being demanding and be regarded as a problem.

The nurse may mean a number of things when she calls a patient demanding. She may be saying that he wants too much of her time or is actually taking up too much of it; that he is asking for too much attention; that he is making too many requests or asking too many questions. When a nurse says a patient is demanding, she also means that in her present nursing situation she cannot give the patient what he is asking for. That is, she cannot fulfill his demands in view of the number of patients that have to be cared for, the personnel available, her other duties, and her own inclinations and desires.

When a situation arises in which the patient is demanding and the nurse feels "put upon," it is easy to say that the patient's need to be demanding is *his problem*. This is true only in part. From our point of view his demandingness is a problem situation that the nurse and patient create and maintain by their participation with each other. It is not only a problem the patient "has," in the sense that his demands arise from his "need to be demanding"; his demands also arise from the responses of personnel and their relations with him. We know from experience that with some nurses' responses the patient's demands will increase; with others, they will decrease. Thus, the nurse can try to find out how she contributes to an increase or continuation of the patient's demands and how she might deal with the patient to help him give them up.

STAFF REACTIONS TO THE PATIENT'S DEMANDS

It is fairly common for a nurse to react to a patient's excessive demands with impatience or anger. If these feelings are strong, the nurse may have an impulse to stop the demands forcibly or to get away from the patient in order not to hear them. Or the nurse may meet the demands in such a way that the patient realizes she is not interested in meeting them and is only doing so because it is part of her job. These reactions indicate that the nurse feels that the patient is imposing on her, that he "shouldn't be making so many demands," that his behavior is unacceptable to her. With these feelings the nurse is likely to respond to the patient in a way that is not satisfying to him. Because of this response the patient may become more demanding and a situation may be created that is unpleasant and unsatisfactory for both patient and nurse. As an illustration of this we present a ward group discussing a patient's demands.

HEAD NURSE: I'd like to talk about Miss Bell's demands and our experience with the best way of handling them.

MISS ADAMS: The other day when I brought her an ashtray she demanded any number of things. She asked me to get the card table, typewriter, and stationery and envelopes. Well, I had just about reached the limit and I was getting more and more annoyed. Then she told me exactly where she wanted everything put—in the exact position. Then she asked for a cigarette. The more annoyed I became the more demands she made.

DR. HILL: Do you think she could have been so anxious that she didn't know what she wanted?

MISS ADAMS: It may be that she was uncomfortable about something and didn't know just what to do to occupy herself or to relieve some of the feelings she had.

MR. LEWIS: Well, last evening she got to the point where she wanted so much—nuts, this and that kind of candy—that I tried to cut her off, but she just went on asking for things.

With another patient there was a similar problem:

MISS ADAMS: Mrs. Dennis' demands went on all day long. We never could satisfy her. She would stop first one nurse and then another, but we couldn't do anything exactly the way she wanted it done. I became so irritated and angry with her.

MISS BROWN: When this started in the morning, where was the patient and what were you doing?

MISS ADAMS: The patient was standing at the food truck. We had taken her tray to her room. We were busy serving the other breakfast trays.

MISS BROWN: Did the patient know you had served her tray?

MISS ADAMS: I don't know whether she did or not. She asked for coffee. I got it for her. Then she said she wanted the coffer hotter. I went to heat it up. Then she wanted cream and sugar, but I couldn't get it right for her. She asked other students, too. We got fed up with her because we couldn't do anything to please her all day long. By the end of the day we were all irritated with her.

MRS. COLT: She stopped everybody and seemed to get more frantic all the time. We just couldn't seem to please her.

The nurse's annoyance and anger with the patient's requests seem so frequently to perpetuate the demands that it is important to understand what happens in these situations. The more frustrated and unfulfilled the patient feels because of the nurse's actions and feelings, the more demanding he gets. The more demanding the patient gets, the more annoyed and angry the nurse becomes, making it more difficult for her to meet the patient's demands. Thus, a cycle is continued in which the patient is being demanding because he is frustrated and unfulfilled, and the nurse is not responsive to the patient's demands and is not fulfilling his needs because he increases her anger and annoyance. As part of this cycle, by becoming angry or annoyed the nurse withdraws her attention from the patient, ceases trying to understand and supply what he is asking for, and instead becomes involved with and focuses on her own feelings. Because of this, it is difficult to focus on and attend to the patient. We do not mean to imply that the nurse should not have these feelings; ordinarily, she will. When they are present the nurse can recognize them for what they are and then perhaps go on from this recognition to determine what the patient wants and how she can best meet these wants.

There are other reactions on the part of the nurse that seem to get in her way in dealing most appropriately with patients' excessive requests. One of these is the nurse's attitude that the patient is trying to be manipulative or to take advantage of her. She may be afraid that by meeting the patient's numerous requests she will be "indulging him too much" or "giving in to him." This is illustrated in the following situation in which a number of nurses are discussing Miss Jeliffe, a new nurse.

> MISS ADAMS: She [Miss Jeliffe] is going to have a rough time up there. She didn't think we should cater to Joan [a patient]. She won't do it because she doesn't want Joan to think she can get the better of her. She thought we weren't helping the patient by catering to her.
> MISS BROWN: She seems to be quite rigid.
> MISS ADAMS: She said she would just tell Joan off if she came asking her for so many things. I told her I didn't think it would help. I gave her examples of people who had tried it and explained how everyone ended up furious, with Joan making more demands and getting more upset. She couldn't see that we were helping the patients any by giving in to them.
> MRS. COLT: I watched her yesterday with Joan. She was doing the same old thing that increases Joan's demandingness and irritation. Joan would ask her for something and she wouldn't respond to her. Joan would holler, "Do you hear me?" and Jeliffe would still ignore her. It just drove Joan to a frenzy.
> MISS ADAMS: When she said that by giving in to Joan's demands we were not helping her at all, I tried to explain to her the struggle we had had before, and to show her how by meeting Joan's demands we had made them practically die out.

What seems to happen in such situations is that the nurse reacts in an intensely personal way. She experiences the patient's demands as a personal struggle between herself and him. She then focuses on what she believes the patient is "trying to do *against* her," rather than on "What does the patient need?" and "What is he trying to communicate by his request?"

Also important is the nurse's resentment of the manner in which the patient makes the request. The nurse may say that the patient is "too haughty," "too bossy," "He thinks he's a king the way he orders everyone around," or "He treats you like a servant." In effect, the nurse feels that way because the patient's manner is a threat to her self-esteem. She feels he does not respect her but instead looks down upon her, and that he is contemptuous and "pushes her around." If the nurse continues to feel this way, she may become punishing, retaliatory, or rejecting in her attitude toward and treatment of the patient and may thereby increase his demands and disturbance.

There are other ways in which the patient makes the nurse feel insecure and resentful, and because of this resentment and insecurity the nurse is unable to see how desperate the patient is.

MISS ADAMS: The problem with Mrs. James is that she makes constant demands on the personnel—first, of the person in charge, and then she drags everybody else into it. She always has some vital problem that cannot wait more than two seconds to be discussed.

MISS BROWN: A lot of us feel that she's just trying to suck us dry. It seems that there isn't enough that we can give her, her demands are unlimited. And she just hangs on so that I want to run.

SOCIOLOGIST: Does everyone react the same way? Do you all feel annoyed and uncomfortable and want to run away from her? And is this feeling constant, or does it change?

MISS ADAMS: She's very wearing.

MRS. COLT: I can take her for ten or fifteen-minute periods, then I have to leave. She's such a leech when she becomes upset and demanding, I'm about ready to explode when I'm done with her. On the other hand, if we leave her alone or ignore her she just gets more upset and demanding. But she drains you dry, so that you can't be with her long.

MISS DEAN: Sometimes she's so desperate when she screams for you to stay with her. She just clings to you. At times I've been able to calm her and talk with her. Then I don't have so much resentment.

SOCIOLOGIST: There's a great difference between seeing her as a pest and seeing her as a desperate person, as a sick woman whose only way of asking for help is the demanding way.

MR. LEWIS: Sometimes I've been able to talk to her and reassure her, and she'll quiet down in her demands.

SOCIOLOGIST: I think that's important. She seems to be asking for the reassurance that somebody will be around to help her.

MISS ADAMS: It's hard to give it to her, because she gets under your skin the way she hangs on to you.

SOCIOLOGIST: I think we have to recognize how angry she makes us and go on from there; we can't control it. Once we accept our anger, work it out or ride it out, we might be able to figure out something that will help her.

MISS BROWN: We get worn out by her and find her so difficult that we can't meet her demands and then she feels rejected. She doesn't realize that by making demands the way she does she makes it difficult for us to meet them.

In the example given above the nurses are struggling with their antagonistic feelings toward the patient. They recognize, on the one hand, that these feelings do not help them meet the patient's demands, and, on the other, that they do have these antagonistic feelings. We have found that in the process of expressing themselves and talking over their reactions, nurses come to be able to deal with their feelings and with the patient more effectively. Out of the discussion comes better understanding of their own feelings and of the patient's need for reassurance and support.

Continuing to refuse or ignore a patient's requests may make him more demanding. With some patients, however, it may contribute to withdrawal or greater muteness. Repeated rebuffs may force the patient to shut himself up, withdraw into a shell, and avoid relations with others. He may then be less demanding and, therefore, easier to deal with, but encouraging him in such withdrawal may also perpetuate his illness. The recognition of this possibility is expressed by personnel in a discussion of Miss Bell, who had been asking incessantly for cigarettes.

MR. LEWIS: You know, there was a time when she didn't smoke.

MISS ADAMS: There was a time when she didn't eat, either. During that time she wouldn't open her eyes.

HEAD NURSE: That's the thing that worries me. She may be demanding now, but she was catatonic previously. If we cut her off too much we might be encouraging her to go back to that stage. She might feel, "If you won't give me anything, I don't want anything." Then she becomes a lump of flesh without any movement. I suppose if we restrict her too much there is always the possibility that she might go back to that stage, especially since she's been there before.

MR. SHERMAN: If you give the patients everything they want, everything they ask for, it still doesn't seem as though they are satisfied.

MISS BROWN: If we gave them everything they ask for, it would be impossible up there.

HEAD NURSE: Well, you can't give them everything they ask for, because some of the things we can't give them anyway, and there are definite limits on our time. But we could show them we're really interested in meeting their requests within the limits of our capabilities.

There are two concerns that are common among nurses with reference to a patient's excessive requests. One is that the more a patient's requests are fulfilled the more they will increase. The other is that the nurse may have to grant *all* of the patient's requests for a long period of time before his demands will decrease. With reference to the first concern, there may be times when a patient's requests come fast and furiously and meeting one seems to encourage him to make another. On the one hand, if the nurse could accept the demands during these periods she might discover that the periods are only temporary, and that the patient gives up his demands when he no longer feels he has to fight to have his needs fulfilled. Once the patient develops some conviction that the nurse is interested in fulfilling his requests, he no longer needs to be demanding. On the other hand, if the nurse becomes annoyed, reluctant, withholding, or strict with the patient, he tends to increase his demands.

With reference to the second concern, it is quite impossible for a nurse to fulfill all the requests of a patient. But it is not necessary to do so. All the nurse may have to do is listen to these requests, show an interest in trying to understand them, and determine what needs the patient is trying to have fulfilled through them. If the nurse can show such consideration for a patient's requests, tries to respond to them within the limits of the situation, and gives reasons when they cannot be met, she may discover that the patient quickly gives up his excessive demands.

If the nurse can see the patient's demands as one of the forms his mental illness is taking at this time, she may be able to look beyond her irritation, resentment, and annoyance to the meaning of the demands for the patient, to the needs that motivate them, and to her own part in maintaining or changing this behavior.

MEANING OF THE PATIENT'S DEMANDS TO HIM

We have found that once the nurse gets an inkling of the significance of a patient's excessive requests, her anger and antagonism decrease and become less of a factor in her relations with the patient. She becomes more interested in finding out what the patient's needs are and how she can meet them. Thus, it is important to ask: What is the patient trying to communicate through his demands? What could these demands possibly mean to him? A continuation of the conference about Miss Bell suggests that the patient's demands may be related to a need for attention and a great fear of being deprived.

> MR. LEWIS: One day when she got angry at me she said that she didn't get enough attention and this was one way of getting it—by being demanding and irritable.
>
> MISS COLT: I think Miss Bell is a person who doesn't feel important enough in her own right. She doesn't think her needs will be satisfied. She has a feeling she's going to be deprived because she isn't deserving or isn't important. Her demands grow out of her fear that she won't get anything.
>
> HEAD NURSE: She doesn't expect that anybody is going to give her anything. She has to ask for everything she's going to get and she better keep asking fast and furiously.
>
> SOCIOLOGIST: It all depends on how you regard her. If you look upon her as the kind of person who is trying to annoy you, then it's very difficult to give her much. But if you look upon her as somebody who is quite lost and very anxious and fearful about the world, then it's much easier to try to give her something. If you could see her as in great need, rather than feeling attacked by her or looking upon her as somebody who's trying to make you uncomfortable, then you might be able to help her.

In other instances, a patient's requests may be related to her feelings of helplessness, even though her manner appears to be domineering.

> MR. LEWIS: Yesterday Alice asked me for an ashtray that was quite within reach. It was right by her but she insisted I get it for her. I did because somehow I felt it was important to do it.

Miss Adams: It's hard to realize how helpless and desperate she is. When she commands you, you feel as though she's ordering you around, but inside she is very weak, frightened, and terrified, as if she were nothing. One way she can feel like something is by shouting and having people jump to meet her demands. When she demands something she acts as though you were dirt under her feet, and we feel angry because it does something to our own self-esteem.

Mr. Sherman: My attitude toward her changed the day she asked me for something and I wouldn't give it to her. She cried and I really felt sorry for her.

Miss Adams: When we get hard on her and restrict her, she becomes more frightened and helpless. We forget how helpless she really is when we get so involved with ourselves.

Sometimes a patient by her repeated, insistent demands reveals the extent of her desperation and need for an interested response from the nurse.

Miss Adams: There is one thing about Mrs. Carton that is upsetting to us. She keeps asking us to tell her what to do. She tries to put you into the position of making every decision for her. She's extremely dependent and leaves you drained.

Miss Brown: She just seems to suck you dry with her demands.

Miss Adams: Like this evening—just when I was ready to leave she had something of major importance to discuss with me. It's always something that has to be decided at once and can't wait until tomorrow.

Miss Brown: I just feel depleted when I spend a little time with her.

Sociologist: It seems that she's desperate about forming a relationship, so she goes on in this fashion. She has told me that she's so lonesome, that she's never had anybody or had anything.

Mrs. Colt: Yet she sets it up in such a way that she drives you away with her clinging and demanding.

Miss Adams: You get a feeling of real desperation from her. I want to do something for her and yet she drives me away when she's so insistent and won't let go of me.

Sociologist: She clings to the students and screams and yells so for them when they're not there that they just want to run and hide from her. So far she's chased almost everybody away. She wants so desperately to draw people toward her, yet she chases them away.

Miss Adams: She seems to be terribly frightened when she clings that way.

In situations such as the above the nurse clearly recognizes the patient's desperation and is made anxious by her desperate plea. The nurse feels a demand is made on her to "do something," yet she does not know what to do or how to do it. The more desperate the patient becomes, the more helpless and the less able the nurse may become to cope with his demands. The nurse feels the patient's needs to be so overwhelming that she does not know where to start in trying to meet them. Perhaps the nurse can start by recognizing the patient's extreme anxiety—that behavior which tells the nurse "something is wrong"—and that the demands stem in part from this anxiety. She also might notice how the patient makes her anxious. With some awareness of her own as well as the patient's anxiety, she might try to focus her attention on relating to the patient in a reassuring way. In addition, it is important to respond to the patient immediately—respond, that is, by indicating recognition of his plight and showing concern about it. The desperate, demanding patient is asking for someone to help him here and now. Ignoring him or putting him off may reinforce his despair about ever having his needs met.

From one point of view a patient's constant requests may be looked upon as having positive aspects. Through them he might be telling the nurse something she can listen to and try to understand.

DR. HILL: When you say a patient is demanding, do you mean he interacts more with the people around him?

MISS ADAMS: No, he is just making constant requests for something.

DR. HILL: But that is a type of communication with others. It seems to me that when you say a patient is more demanding, you mean he is more alert to what goes on and more in contact with the people around him and making the contact in the only way that is available to him. It often looks hostile and we call it demanding. "Demanding" is very much in the listener's ears, and it is one way of approaching another person when you're afraid that your needs aren't going to be satisfied. I'd rather have a patient demanding than withdrawn.

DR. LYONS: I think there may be two reasons why patients in our hospital are more demanding. We encourage communication here; we try to get the patients to speak up and speak out—we try to get them to express themselves. The second reason is that we try to meet a patient's individual needs, and the patient feels that there is this possibility here.

MISS BROWN: If we could take care of patients' demands a little more spontaneously and easily, they probably wouldn't become excessive.

Patients may use their demands as a way of relating to another person and keep repeating them in order to maintain the relationship.

INSTRUCTOR: Do you remember when we were talking about Mrs. Dennis and her difficulties with the coffee? Maybe the specific things she was asking for, the cream and sugar for instance, were not the important things. It may be that the patient has a hard time relating to people and that she is attempting to relate with you through the coffee situation. You seem to keep putting your emphasis only on the coffee situation or the other things she asks for and not on the fact that she might be trying to establish a relationship with you through asking for these things.

Let's see how we can go about understanding this. The nurse begins by getting irritated and says, "No matter what I do, I can't satisfy this woman." So the next step is to ask why. And maybe it's because the coffee isn't the important thing. Now I don't know whether this will change anything or not, but you might try it: When the patient comes to the food truck tomorrow, you could say, "Hi, why don't you sit down there. I have some coffee for you. We can talk while I'm serving the trays. Then you can have yours here or in your room if you like. While you're having breakfast I'll sit down and have something with you." Of course, there might be other ways of doing it, but let's see what happens if you try this one.

The patient may use her demands as a way of maintaining some contact with reality and as a way of getting outside her own private world.

MISS ADAMS: When Miss Howard asks me to do something and I can't do it, I point out to her that I'm doing something for someone else. She'll accept the fact that you can't do something for her on the spot. This makes it easier for her to accept a delay. The other thing is that she is a patient who is autistic most of the time. When she comes into reality for a few minutes and we aren't there, I can see how she feels we don't do enough for her. I don't think she's fully aware of how much we do for her.

MISS BROWN: That reminds me of Miss Knowles. She was pre-occupied most of the time with her own little world. Every few min-utes she'd interrupt her fantasies and ask for a cigarette. For a brief minute she made a contact with the nurse and then went back to her own world. This asking for a cigarette so frequently struck us as very demanding, but as soon as we recognized that she was keeping in contact with reality or with someone else through these demands, it was much easier for us to accept them.

We have seen ways in which the feelings about and reactions to the patient influence his demands: rejection and denial tend to increase them and interest in meeting the patient's needs tends to decrease them. We also have had some indication of the meaning and significance of these demands. They are indicators of the patient's anxiety and desperation, and at the same time they are attempts to relate with others. It now remains for us to describe some successful resolutions of situations in which the patient was demanding.

DEALING WITH PATIENT DEMANDS

As a result of the discussion of Miss Bell and subsequent similar discussions, personnel had a different view of her as well as a better understanding of the significance of her requests. They changed their attitude toward the patient. Instead of being an-noyed they developed a genuine desire to meet her requests as rapidly and adequately as possible, trying to anticipate them. At a conference they report on the change in the patient's behavior.

HEAD NURSE: What has happened to Miss Bell's demands?
MR. LEWIS: Well, she hasn't been too demanding these days. When she asks for anything I give it to her if I can. Sometimes if I'm busy and she keeps demanding something from the kitchen, I tell her to come and get it, and she'll come.
HEAD NURSE: I'm wondering if the fact that we talked about her and got an idea of what might be a good way to handle her helped; that is, talking about trying to meet her demands and anticipate them. After the meeting Miss Bell didn't make me nearly so mad. I didn't mind doing things for her, and a lot of other people felt the same way. In the last few days we've had no difficulty with her being demanding.

One of the nurses followed the instructor's suggestion that she offer Mrs. Dennis some coffee before she asked for it. When the nurse did this, Mrs. Dennis was less demanding. Miss Adams reported that the patient was sick in bed with a cold, and that she had taken coffee to her room before breakfast was served and *before* the patient asked for it. She also indicated to the patient that she would sit with her while she drank the coffee.

> INSTRUCTOR: What happened?
> MISS ADAMS: She just took the coffee and seemed pleased that I wanted to stay.
> INSTRUCTOR: Did she complain about the sugar and cream not being right?
> MISS ADAMS: No. I just put cream and sugar in and decided if she didn't say anything about it, it was all right. She didn't gripe about anything, and she was really pleased to have me with her; she was so different from yesterday when her demands made everyone angry with her.

An aide indicates how her changed attitude led to a change in her own behavior and to a change in the patient's behavior, in the direction of greater mutual satisfaction.

> MRS. ROGERS: I used to dislike Joan so when she made those demands. I just couldn't stand her. She made me so angry because of the contemptuous way she treated me when demanding something. Then I began to think, "What if I were in her place and needed all these things?" She really thinks she needs them very much. So I started getting things for her before she asked for them and she became much nicer and less demanding, and now I feel much better about her.
> SUPERVISOR: What changed your attitude?
> MRS. ROGERS: One evening she had me going in circles with her demands. Once when I went into her room, she touched me on the shoulder and said, "Give me six pieces of tissue." Her touch on my shoulder and the way she said it made me feel at the time that she just seemed lost.

In the following example one nurse's response to a patient's demands is in marked contrast to that of the rest of the staff, with a marked difference in response from the patient.

> Mrs. Carton had been demanding all day. As soon as any of the personnel came near her she would ask them to stay with her, to

bring her something from the kitchen, to answer some question she was struggling with, or to instruct her how to do something. Personnel had become exasperated and were trying to avoid her. If she did catch them, they would either put her off or ignore her request. It just seemed that they could not do enough for her, and whatever they did only brought on additional requests. Miss Jones [a nurse on the evening shift] came on duty and heard what had been happening with Mrs. Carton. She was calling from her room, trying to attract someone's attention. Miss Jones went immediately to her room and said very sincerely, "Mrs. Carton, I'll be in the office and you can call me anytime you want to." The patient called her once or twice and the nurse responded immediately. But after that Mrs. Carton made scarcely any requests the rest of the evening.

What happened here? There was no magic in the nurse's words. Rather, the nurse accepted the patient's asking for things, recognizing that this was something the patient had to do. Having accepted it, the nurse by her manner and subsequent response conveyed this acceptance to the patient and with it genuine concern for her and desire to meet her needs as best she could. Once the patient is reassured that the nurse wants to meet her needs, she no longer has to keep insisting that her needs be met. It is only when she senses opposition, reluctance, or rejection that she struggles for recognition. The decrease in the patient's requests through this kind of experience is different from the patient's desisting from making requests because she is afraid she will be punished, or giving up with the hopeless feeling that no one is really interested in her. Here, the nurse responded to the patient's general need for reassurance and for having someone attend to her at that particular time.

Another conference shows the importance of the nurse's interest in and anticipation of the patient's requests in making the patient more comfortable.

> MISS ADAMS: One of Joan's problems was her demandingness. For a while she made about four demands a minute in a loud, screeching voice until people around her were just frantic. Personnel were very much annoyed with her and resistant to meeting her demands, and the problem increased considerably. We had several ward meetings about this. We finally got around to seeing that maybe it was her need to be recognized as a person that caused her to be so demanding

and this was the only way she knew how to get recognition. So we decided that we would try to meet her demands, even go a step further and guess at what they might be, and give her something before she asked. Some of the personnel were reluctant to do this but agreed to go along with us. Everyone got cigarettes for her and other such things. Within a short time her demands died down, not entirely but to a great degree. Just recently we had two people come to the ward who could not see eye to eye with us in this. They had a great deal of feeling about meeting these demands. The next two days Joan was practically in a panic. She was screaming as if her life depended on the particular thing she was requesting. I think this is pretty good evidence that meeting her demands was important to her, because it meant that people cared about her.

HEAD NURSE: The outstanding characteristics of patients like Joan is that they feel so deprived, and they're so empty in terms of having anything. It would really, I think, be quite a shock to them if somebody were to come and say, "What can I get you?" instead of their having to ask somebody different each time to get them something. I think you might ask when you pass a patient, "Is there anything you want, is there anything I can get you, is there anything you need?"

MISS ADAMS: I think you can take it a step further than that. I mean, I think you can actually get the patient something.

HEAD NURSE: Even before you ask her?

MISS ADAMS: Just go to her. This works very well with Joan when you take her a cigarette, some tissues, or a cracker, for example.

SOCIOLOGIST: What sort of response do you get?

MISS ADAMS: Well, at first she looked rather startled. She doesn't any more, because I've taken her things every once in a while. With Miss Jackson, this was the only way I could get anywhere with her for a long time—by taking her something at half-hour intervals.

One difficulty a nurse might encounter in anticipating a patient's demands is that she does not know what the patient wants. In these circumstances if the nurse can give something of herself to the patient—her time, attention, and interest—he might understand that the nurse is not reluctant to fulfill his demand, but that she does not understand what he is asking for. The nurse might help the patient see her lack of understanding by simply stating, "I want to get you what you need, but I don't know what it is, and you'll have to help me figure it out."

This final example shows the interrelation between the nurse's reactions, her understanding of the significance of the patient's requests, and the way she deals with the patient.

HEAD NURSE: Miss Jackson's reputation on the ward was that of a demanding patient. Nurses thought that they simply couldn't meet her demands because they were so frequent and so unreasonable.

SOCIOLOGIST: It seems to me that the ward personnel missed the point here. The fact is that Miss Jackson wants to relate with someone; this is the only way she now knows how to do it.

HEAD NURSE: But we all experienced her as demanding.

SOCIOLOGIST: I didn't mean to say that you're not supposed to experience irritation with her demands—that's unavoidable, but can you go further and recognize that you are missing the patient's need? I don't think the nurse can be superhuman. It is natural for her to be irritated, but once having the irritation, can she recognize it and go on to say, "Something is wrong here: the patient is wanting something. I wonder if I can find out what it is and give it to her?" Staying away from her or ignoring her because of one's irritation doesn't meet her needs.

HEAD NURSE: I think most of us recognize that by her demands the patient was trying to relate to us, but it's the way she made her requests, and the repetitiveness and rapidity of them that made some of us withdraw from her. It wasn't until I talked with you that I recognized this withdrawal. I was quite convinced we were waiting on her hand and foot. I started to become aware that I responded to the patient by putting her off, muttering something in response, and then forgetting about it. When I became aware of this, we worked out a plan whereby demands that could be met would be fulfilled immediately and those that could not, such as "Will you let me out of the hospital?" would be answered, "No," directly, and then she would be told why. Finally, we tried to anticipate some of her requests before she made them. After we tried this approach for awhile the number of her requests went way down. Personnel began devoting more time to her and they were more comfortable with her. Also, we found out something that was very important: Miss Jackson made these numerous requests when she became anxious and needed the security of somebody around her. She couldn't say what was bothering her, so she would just go on making one request after another. The requests seemed unnecessary to us; we were so busy and we became irritable and resentful. This only increased her anxiety, and her requests became sharper and more demanding. We responded with more irritation and anxiety, and we didn't recognize our own withdrawal and our ignoring of her requests.

SOCIOLOGIST: At the beginning we misunderstood what the patient was trying to do. We regarded her requests as a pain in the neck, instead of recognizing that this was her way of trying to relate to us. Once we realized this, the demands could be reduced and satisfaction came to the patient and staff. But at the time this was the only way the patient could show her need. This is what it means to be mentally ill—not to be able to use what is appropriate, or to use direct or efficient ways of forming a human relationship and satisfying your needs. The patient uses an indirect way instead—a way that is apt not to bring her what she wants. Once we understand what the patient is communicating and go toward her, the pattern of demandingness almost disappears. In addition, we become more comfortable, more accepting of the patient, and more able to relate to her. Then we experience satisfaction in understanding and meeting her needs.

One point in the last example needs to be elaborated, the withdrawal of the nurse from the patient. We indicated previously that at times when a patient's demands are desperate and anxiety-laden, the nurse will also become anxious. *Under the pressure of this anxiety she may actually not hear the patient's pleas or requests for help,* or she may physically hear them and automatically ignore them. The nurse has to defend herself against the anxiety created by the patient's desperation. If she faces up to the anxiety each time, she may find the stress too great; therefore, occasionally she has to "block out" the desperation in the patient's request or "not hear" the request itself. One of the ways of doing this is to label the patient "demanding," eliminate him from her awareness, and thereby avoid listening to or trying to deal with his requests.

We have suggested that the nurse try to discover what her reactions are to a patient's excessive requests and how her reactions affect the patient's further demands. We do not mean to imply that limits should not be placed on a patient. In some circumstances, not fulfilling a particular demand the patient is making may be of benefit to him. We will discuss the setting of limits on a patient in a later section. Here we suggest that the nurse try to understand some of the meanings that might underlie patient demands. With this recognition and understanding she might be able to participate more appropriately and effectively with the demanding patient.

From our discussion it is perhaps a little clearer why we said earlier that demandingness is a problem created by patient and personnel as they participate with each other. On the one hand, the patient is demanding because of his needs and because of the nurse's reactions to his demands. On the other hand, the nurse's feelings, reactions, and understanding influence the way she responds to the patient and thus influence whether he will continue to be demanding or not. If the nurse is indifferent to the patient's demands, he may have to continue them until something changes in the situation. When the nurse conveys an attitude of concern for the patient's needs and tries to understand, accept, and meet his demands, we have found that demanding patients often give up their demandingness, with increased comfort and satisfaction resulting for both patients and staff. We should emphasize, however, that our purpose has not been to help the nurse prohibit the patient's demands or silence the patient. Eliminating the patient's demands in this way may only result in the appearance of other symptoms, such as withdrawal or assaultiveness. Rather, our interest has been to help the nurse use the patient's demands as a vehicle for establishing a better relationship between them, *that is, relating to the patient around his demands in such a way that his security and self-esteem are increased and satisfaction is derived by him from the relationship. Through this improved relationship it may become unnecessary for him to continue to be demanding.*

<small>«</small> 4 <small>»</small>

The Patient Is Withdrawn

IN a previous chapter we described the assaultive patient—one who comes *toward* the personnel, if only to attack them. The subject of this chapter is the withdrawn patient—one who *stays away from* the nurse, even though this means that some of his important needs are not fulfilled.

The patient who is silent, apathetic, keeps to himself, and does not "bother" anyone is not a problem for the nurse in the sense that he "makes trouble" for her. However, withdrawn patients are serious problems from another point of view. The patient's withdrawal may be a significant part of his mental illness; that is, his avoidance of people and tendency to remain isolated may be one of his primary difficulties in living with others. If he continues to be withdrawn he continues his mental illness.

While they are withdrawn, patients appear to be concentrating on and preoccupied with their own inner world. This self-preoccupation makes it easy for the nurse to look upon the patient's withdrawal as something "inside" the patient, about which she can do very little. On the other hand, she might see the patient's withdrawal as a response to those around him. Our view is that both factors are present. What goes on inside the patient is influenced by other people's activities with him; at the same time, what goes on inside him influences the behavior of others. We will focus primarily on how nurses might contribute to a patient's tendency to withdraw and perhaps reinforce it, and on the ways they might help the patient carry on relations with others. In order to do this we will discuss what withdrawal might mean to a patient, what it means to the nurse, and some ways in which nurses relate to withdrawn patients.

It is important to distinguish between solitude and withdrawal. In solitude one takes time out to be alone, to think, to contemplate events that have occurred, or to become reacquainted with oneself and the changes that have happened in one's life. One temporarily removes oneself from relations with others. But in a withdrawn state the patient is constantly by himself and away from others. Only rarely does he associate with anyone on his own initiative. When someone approaches him, he appears to be reluctant and unwilling to have anything to do with him. In extreme withdrawal, personnel actually have to force the patient into some contact with others (for example, by tube-feeding him) in order to keep him alive.

As an example of a withdrawn patient we present a description of Miss Black, as reported by a nurse.

> MISS CROFT: Day after day Miss Black does the same thing. She spends most of the time lying on her bed. She won't get off it by herself, and we have a hard time getting her off to take her to the bathroom or to give her a bath. She resists us when we try to get her off. She seems so scared when one of us comes near her; she shrinks into herself, turns her back on us, or becomes frozen. She won't respond when we speak to her, and when we look directly at her she looks away and becomes more frightened. Whenever we do get her out of her room she'll run right back to her bed. She won't talk to anyone, not even to other patients, and when you come near her, she acts as if you weren't there. When she knows you are watching her, she'll look blank and stare at the wall. When she doesn't see you and doesn't know you are looking at her, she seems alert to what's going on.

The sameness of the routine and the lack of variation in the patient's behavior made the nurse feel that it was almost impossible to change the patient or help her move in another direction.

Some withdrawn patients may be more active physically than Miss Black but still spend the major portion of their time away from others, in self-seclusion or isolation. For us a withdrawn patient is one who is silent almost all the time he is near another person. He talks only occasionally, takes little initiative with others, and shows little overt responsiveness to approaches from others. The patient may ignore the nurse when she talks to him, or he may just stare at her. Some withdrawn patients sit in the day room for many hours without moving but are alert to their surroundings. Others stretch out on the floor, apparently oblivious to the activity around them or the movements made toward them. Some do not seem to care what happens and give the impression that they do not have the energy or cannot put forth the effort to "bother with anyone else." By avoiding others, the withdrawn patient denies himself the opportunity to share experiences with them and to develop satisfying relationships with them. Under these circumstances the patient cannot correct some of his misinterpretations about others; he cannot benefit from what others have to offer him; he cannot change his preoccupation with himself; nor can he modify his thoughts and feelings about "what is real and what isn't." Since the kind of experiences the patient needs in order to improve can come only from continuing relations with others, it is important for the nurse to help bring about such relations. That is, she can help to make it unnecessary for the patient to continue to be withdrawn. This does not mean that the patient should be "pushed into" activity, that is, urged, cajoled, or physically forced. Nor can we state specifically "what the nurse should do" in order to stimulate and activate a patient. This is a matter of discovery for each nurse to make with each patient with whom she deals.

What are some of the feelings of patients who show a marked tendency to withdraw from others? These patients might be shy and frightened of other people. They maintain an air of aloofness because they feel uncertain and uncomfortable with others. Their detached manner or attitude might give the nurse the impression that they do not need her or want her around. If a patient continues this cold, indifferent response to her, the nurse might become convinced that he does not want to have anything to do with her. But this is only part of the patient's feelings. At the same time that he may want to avoid and shun others because of the pain he has experienced from them, another part of him very much wants some relationship with the nurse. He may even feel that he needs the nurse desperately, but he may be unable to show his need to the nurse or even to recognize the intensity with which he wants recognition and attention from others. The patient's suspicions and distrust of another's motives stand in the way of his revealing and expressing his need for companionship. In addition, the withdrawn patient may feel hopeless and discouraged about being able to form a satisfying relationship with another, expecting to be misunderstood, to be unable to communicate, or to be treated with contempt and rejected for his inadequacies.

The Nurse's Contribution to Patient Withdrawal

If a patient continues to be withdrawn for a long period of time, it is likely that some nurses will tend to avoid him, either deliberately or without being aware of it. If the patient's and nurse's avoidance of each other continues over a period of time, a situation of *mutual withdrawal* may be established. In this situation the patient's withdrawal is perpetuated and reinforced by the nurse's avoidance of him. It is as if the patient were acting on the idea (not deliberately, but perhaps in spite of himself) "if you will not have anything to do with me, I'll ignore you and act as if you didn't exist." The patient's resentment and pain, which result from being avoided by the nurse, only "drive him" further into his shell. The nurse cannot expect the patient to take the first step in changing this situation of mutual withdrawal. She must take the initiative in noticing her own avoidance, then changing it, and, finally, encouraging and helping the patient to give up his withdrawal. Therefore, it becomes important for the nurse to discover and recognize the ways in which her own feelings about the patient prevent her from helping him with his withdrawal.

The *anxiety or discomfort* the nurse feels in being with a withdrawn patient seems to play an important part in later keeping her away from the patient. In the situation described below the head nurse and the sociologist are talking about a nurse, Mrs. Ives, who has been trying to spend some time with a withdrawn patient but has had a great deal of difficulty doing so. The nurse stays with the patient a few minutes, leaves her, and does not go

back. Usually, she finds something else to do instead of going back
to the patient.

> HEAD NURSE: Mrs. Ives has been having a hard time staying with
> Katherine lately. She feels the patient is scorning her by her stony
> silence. Mrs. Ives is discouraged about being able to make any con-
> tact with her. She says she's very uncomfortable with Katherine.
> SOCIOLOGIST: She can't take it?
> HEAD NURSE: I told her the important thing is to keep going back
> so that Katherine will know that she's really interested. I said, "The
> patient is frightened because all her life people have shown little in-
> terest in her, and when they did they soon left. If you keep going
> back to her, it might take a little time for her to be convinced, but
> she will respond. If you persist with her she'll do more with you."
> Mrs. Ives said she would try it. But so far, Katherine just sits with her
> back turned to her, masturbates, and doesn't pay any attention to
> her.
> SOCIOLOGIST: She's a very difficult patient to be with. I've seen
> people go in there intending to stay with her, and in two minutes
> they came flying out; they just couldn't stay there. The only way you
> can stand it is to become very observant and watch the slightest ges-
> ture she makes. Otherwise you'll get very uncomfortable.

What happens in these situations when the nurse becomes
anxious with a patient and then because of her anxiety tends to
avoid him? We are used to having another person respond when
we approach him, and we usually expect a verbal response to our
words. In the illustration above the nurse cannot take the patient's long periods of silence. She has not yet learned to sit in
silence with a patient. In addition, the nurse is made uncomfortable by the patient's apparent lack of interest in her. In these
situations a nurse wants to do something for the patient but is
made to feel unnecessary, incapable of being of use to him now,
and hopeless and helpless about ever being able to help him.
Thus, the patient's silence, his indifference, and his rejection
make the nurse so uncomfortable that she has to leave him. Often
she does not recognize that she is leaving the patient for her own
comfort. She thinks instead that there is something important
that needs to be done, that the patient does not really need her,
or that she can spend her time more profitably elsewhere. When
the nurse has had a few uncomfortable experiences with a with-

drawn patient, she wants to avoid the repetition of these uncomfortable situations, or she avoids them without being aware of it. Therefore, she avoids the patient in anticipation of the anxiety and discomfort she will feel in relating to him. This is a frequent way in which a stable situation of mutual withdrawal comes about. In these situations the nurse expects the patient to be silent, unresponsive, and anxiety-provoking; therefore, she avoids him. In part because he is avoided, the patient avoids contacts with others. He continues to fulfill the nurse's expectations as long as she encourages his withdrawal and does not help him to do something about it.

When a nurse deals with a withdrawn patient, feelings of disappointment, hurt, discouragement, and hopelessness about the patient are bound to arise. Often these feelings, especially if unrecognized, lead to the nurse's avoidance of the patient.

MISS FRY: I've tried to spend some time with Miss Levin [a patient].

SOCIOLOGIST: How did it go?

MISS FRY: She showed a lot of hostility toward me.

SOCIOLOGIST: What did she say or do?

MISS FRY: She said, "Why don't you leave me alone?" I said, "Well, I'm interested in you." She said, "How could you be interested in me when you don't even know me?" I said, "I've become interested in you since I've been acquainted with you on the ward." She said she didn't like to talk to anybody she didn't know. Then she kept quiet and wouldn't have anything more to do with me. There was a long period of silence, and then she pretended to be asleep. I asked her how she felt about my spending time with her. She said, "It annoys me very much."

SOCIOLOGIST: How did you feel about that?

MISS FRY: I was disappointed and hurt by it. She was so hostile in the way she said it. I said, "Would you like me to leave now?" She did not answer, so I just left.

SOCIOLOGIST: Have you been back to see her?

MISS FRY: I can't remember having visited her since then.

Another situation is described below. Here a nurse becomes discouraged in trying to relate to a withdrawn patient.

HEAD NURSE: Have you been spending much time with Alice?

MISS MARKS: I've been sitting with her, but I have the feeling I'm upsetting her rather than helping her. When I tried to read to her, she'd say, "Please leave me alone."

HEAD NURSE: It must be hard for you.

MISS MARKS: It's so easy to get discouraged. Each time I go in to see her it seems harder to reach her than the last time. She lies there as if she were asleep. She won't talk to me, and the least little attempt I make to do anything she just pushes me away. Reading to her doesn't seem to be the thing to do for her right now. I really don't think she likes me.

HEAD NURSE: I don't think that's it. Maybe she's not ready for words right now.

MISS MARKS: I just feel lost when I try to think of things to do for her.

HEAD NURSE: You'll have to think of things on a nonverbal level.

MISS MARKS: I've tried so many things—just sitting there, looking at a magazine with her. Every time I've tried she's pulled away from me. I just feel at a standstill. I no longer know what to do.

Sometimes in a discouraged mood a nurse reveals the effect a withdrawn patient has on her.

MISS MARKS: I thought about going in to see her, but I was too tired and uncomfortable to put up with her silence and rebuffs. She receives me a lot of the time as if I weren't there. I don't think this out consciously, but I feel, "What's the difference if I do go in to see her, she probably won't even realize that I'm there." At times when I sit with her I don't know why I do this because it seems as if she weren't even aware of my existence.

What are some other feelings about and reactions to the patient that lead the nurse to withdraw from him? The nurse may become impatient because she has invested much time and energy in the patient and she sees no change in him. Or her lack of success after repeated attempts to interest him may lead to a persistent discouragement. She may become discouraged because the patient has made some progress and then "slips back." When a nurse has had a good relationship with a patient and he rebuffs and ignores her, she may feel hurt and disappointed. If after repeated attempts to establish a relationship with the patient he shows only contempt for her, the nurse's self-esteem may be lowered. In these instances the nurse may lose interest in the patient, feel hopeless about him, or believe that she cannot help him or is wasting her time with him.

If avoidance of a patient is widespread and persists among the nursing staff as a whole, he may be forgotten, neglected, or overlooked. Under these circumstances, the patient seldom comes to the nurse's attention and rarely enters into her thinking as a source of interest or concern. When the patient is brought to her attention, she may unconsciously dismiss him or quickly forget what she was going to do for him.

A nurse also may contribute to a patient's withdrawal by becoming accustomed to it and not looking upon it as a problem. It is especially easy for the nurse to become accustomed to the patient's withdrawal if none of the other personnel is concerned about it or sees it as a difficulty about which something needs to be done. In these circumstances, the nurse experiences the patient's behavior as his "natural" way of behaving. She unconsciously thinks of him as "that kind of patient," and, therefore, does not have to do anything "about him." She might also feel indifferent and respond to the patient in an automatic, routinized way. This attitude ordinarily goes on without any awareness on her part until the patient gradually disappears into the environment, his withdrawal almost completely unnoticed by her. This inclination unconsciously to acclimate herself to the patient's withdrawal is difficult to recognize, especially when the nurse has a tendency to avoid the patient or when her many other duties do not give her much time to focus on a particular patient who does not bring himself to her attention. In these situations the nurse needs to develop and maintain the awareness that the patient's withdrawal as well as her own is a problem that she must continually try to solve.

There is an idea current among some nursing personnel that certain patients go through cyclical periods and that each phase of the cycle has to run its course before the patient will change his behavior. This conception might be held about a withdrawn patient who has been diagnosed manic-depressive, depressed; his withdrawal might be looked upon as a phase of the cycle about which nothing can be done. With such a conception the nurse contributes to the continuation of the patient's withdrawal by thinking, "He will have to come out of his withdrawn state by himself. No matter what anyone does he has to go through this." The nurse very well might use the idea of the cycle as a rationalization for not doing anything about the withdrawn patient. Our view is that even if there is such a cyclical phase in the patient's illness, the nurse can influence it in important ways by what she does with the patient. She can precipitate one or another phase of it; she can interrupt the phase the patient is in; she can prolong it; or she can help to bring it to a rapid conclusion. This means that the nurse can influence the withdrawn patient in the direction of greater participation with others, or she can help maintain him in his withdrawal. The patient's movement is not dependent only upon what is going on "inside of him" or upon the dictates of a cycle through which he must move. The cycle is flexible. It can be stretched and expanded. It can be changed. The patient is not just a prisoner of some vague force called "a cycle through which his illness must pass."

Another way in which the nurse might encourage or prolong a patient's withdrawal is by rejecting his attempts to relate to others or by ridiculing him for his awkward and inappropriate behavior. As we have indicated previously, the patient's attempts to relate to the nurse might have to take deviant forms. He may try to form a relationship with the nurse through assaultiveness and incontinence, or sexual or demanding behavior. If the nurse cannot accept these ways of relating to her, the patient may become discouraged and feel hopeless about making himself understood or forming any kind of acceptable or satisfying relationship with another. He may give up and become indifferent and apathetic because of the repeated rejections he has suffered from others.

The serious effects on the patient of his continued withdrawal are not obvious but they are nonetheless real. The patient is reinforced in his loneliness, in the feeling that nobody cares, in his self-evaluation that he is of no consequence, in his suspiciousness and distrust of others, and in his resentful view that others are too hurtful even to try to participate with them. As a matter of fact, we have come to believe that prolonged withdrawal on the part of a patient is one of the most important ways in which his mental illness is perpetuated. The nurse can make a significant contribution to the patient's recovery by recognizing situations in which the patient is withdrawn and developing appropriate ways of helping him give up his withdrawal.

HELPING THE WITHDRAWN PATIENT

How can a nurse break through a patient's withdrawal and bring him into greater social participation? As we have indicated before, we do not mean that the nurse should force patients into activity. Rather, we are interested in how the nurse can stimulate and nurture the patient's need and desire for a relationship with another, the circumstances under which the nurse's interest in a withdrawn patient grows and develops, and how a nurse is able to deal with a withdrawn patient in a way that is acceptable to him and encourages his interest in relating to her.

Perhaps the most difficult step in these situations of patient withdrawal is the first one—the recognition that the patient is withdrawn. The nurse has to develop an awareness not only of the fact that the patient is isolating himself and avoiding others, but also of the pattern of activity through which this is done. This means that the nurse tries to discover how the patient blends into the environment and disappears from view, as well as the ways in which she avoids him. One way nursing personnel can discover which patients tend to be overlooked or avoided is to ask themselves in a systematic way questions such as the following: Whose name is likely to be left out when we name the patients on our ward? Who has the fewest or the least informative nursing notes written about him? For which patient are nursing notes approximately the same from day to day? About which patient can we give very little information? Which patients, when they are brought up for discussion, make us evasive and eager to change the subject? Which patients do we want to get away from as fast as we can? With which patients is it most difficult to recall the time we last had a visit? Which patients tend to isolate themselves? Can we recognize how they do this?

It is important to discuss *separately and systematically each patient* on the ward in order to evaluate whether the patient is withdrawn and the extent and nature of his withdrawal. A head nurse, a supervisor, or a doctor can often help the nurse answer these questions by discussing them with her in a detailed way. In addition, if the nurse discusses her feelings and attitudes about a patient and what she observes about herself in relation to him, she might discover when and how the patient arouses her anxiety and makes her eager to stay away from him. These feelings, thoughts, and activities are difficult to recognize because they go on outside the nurse's awareness. To bring them into awareness requires persistence in looking for them and the examination and careful observation of one's inner life and the nature of the relations one carries on with others.

Why is it difficult for a nurse to recognize a patient's or her own withdrawal? We have found that the nurse sometimes feels guilty about neglecting or avoiding a patient. This guilt may arise because she disapproves of herself, thinking she is not a good nurse. In addition, she may feel that the persons in authority will disapprove of her if she overlooks or ignores a patient. In order to avoid the guilt and the experience of disapproval that would come with recognition of her neglect of the patient, she unconsciously fails to see her own and the patient's withdrawal.

Once the nurse has become aware of the patient's and her own withdrawal and the forms they usually take, she can ask herself: What kind of behavior can I undertake at this time that will be acceptable to and appropriate for the patient? For some patients who are verbally as well as physically withdrawn, trying to talk with them is inappropriate because it upsets them and makes them more rejecting of the nurse. For example, Miss Jackson had been seclusive, silent, and in her room for many weeks. When people talked to her she did not respond. An aide reports her visit with the patient.

> MISS BALES: The only thing that succeeds with Miss Jackson is not to say anything. If I sit there and don't say anything, she's fairly comfortable. When I start talking to her, she gets very tense.

SOCIOLOGIST: At this time it seems your relation with her has to be through gestures.

MISS BALES: I've put my arm around her at times, and fixed her pillow. She keeps her eyes closed a lot, but she opens them once in awhile to see if I am there. This shows she's aware of what's going on.

SOCIOLOGIST: You may have to sit with her for a long time before you can do much else.

MISS BALES: The couple of times I pushed her to get out of bed, she got upset.

SOCIOLOGIST: You've got to go at the patient's pace. You have to find out what this pace is and stay with it until she can do something else. Right now, it's just sitting there with her.

For a very withdrawn, silent patient, staying in the room and sitting in silence with him may have to be the first step, and it may have to be continued for some time. The nurse has to rely on her sensitivity to recognize when the patient is ready to participate in another way. Personnel sometimes find it difficult to participate with a patient without talking to him. They think that nothing is happening and that they are wasting their time. In long periods of silence, they become bored and their attention wanders from the patient. If the nurse could observe the patient and herself carefully, she might discover that a great deal happens between them at these times. To discover such activity, she can ask questions such as these about the patient: What does the patient's face tell me? Is his mouth drawn and taut? Is he frowning or smiling? Does he have different kinds of poker faces? If so, what do they indicate? Are his eyes open, closed, flashing, or somber? Is the body relaxed or rigid? Under what circumstances does the patient shift from one position to the other? What are the different ways he lies on the bed? Does he cover his head or his face? Does he face me or turn his back to me? How does he hold his head and arms? Similarly, she could ask about herself: What are my movements and body positions when I am with the patient? Am I tense or relaxed? Do I feel I want to leave the room as soon as I can? What do I convey to the patient about my attitudes toward him? Does he experience me as being interested in him? Does he feel I am uncomfortable and reluctant to stay with him? What is the patient communicating to me in this silence, and what am I telling him?

Not only is it important for the nurse to "take the cue from the patient," but it is also important for her to recognize signs given her by patients who have been isolated for long periods of time that they are ready to come out of their shell. We describe below a situation about a patient whom personnel had not been able to reach for some time. The nurse reports a cue the patient gave that she might be ready for some contact.

> MISS SIMS: Mrs. Trent stuck her head out of the door of her room and caught my eye. She pulled her head right back in again. She didn't expect me to see her do this. I took it as a sign that she might want some company, so I went into her room and said, "I had the feeling you wanted to visit with someone." She didn't say anything, but I sat with her a while. When I left I said, "Perhaps we can talk some time." But that's how she acts. She gives you the tiniest hint and you have to catch on to it.

Once the nurse has become aware of the patient's withdrawal and has initiated a contact, it is important for her to persist in the relationship with the patient. We cannot emphasize sufficiently the importance of coming back regularly to see the patient and not disappointing him when he expects you. If such disappointments do occur, it is important for the nurse to explain to the patient the reason she did not return when she said she would.

At times an object or an activity can be used as a vehicle for forming a relationship with a withdrawn patient. For example, Miss Abel was so shy and frightened of others that she "drew into herself" when someone came near her and she was unresponsive when addressed. An aide was able to enlist her interest and have her stay near him when he offered her colored crayons and helped her use them in a coloring book. On one occasion, he was able to play ball with her. In these situations an activity was the medium through which the aide stimulated the patient's responsiveness and established and maintained a relationship with her.

What are some of the ways in which the nurse can form and maintain a relationship with a withdrawn patient? What are the various processes involved in facilitating the patient's participation? In order to answer these questions, we will trace a relationship between a nurse and patient over a period of time.

Miss Levin is a seclusive patient who has been spending a great deal of time in her room. When personnel approach her, she rejects or ignores them. Miss Harris, a nurse on the ward, has noticed how withdrawn the patient is and has become interested in trying to do something with her. In a discussion with the sociologist Miss Harris gives her initial impressions of Miss Levin and reveals how uncomfortable she is made by the patient's apparent lack of response to and interest in her.

January 6

Miss Harris: When I go in to talk to her I usually get a cold stare, which is very difficult for me to take. When I make rounds she just sits and looks at me. I stand and stare at her, try to make a few comments, and then I leave.

Sociologist: How much of the time is she out of her room?

Miss Harris: About 10 per cent or less.

Sociologist: Does she have any contact with the other patients?

Miss Harris: No, she never approaches them, nor does she approach us. I think she has a great deal of difficulty understanding what we say to her. When I say anything, she just freezes me out.

Sociologist: She's a patient who can be easily ignored because of this response.

Miss Harris: We don't go into her room unless we have to. She won't dress, so we dress her.

Sociologist: She never comes out and asks for anything?

Miss Harris: Just to go to the bathroom. She talks occasionally, usually in a sarcastic way.

The nurse groped for a way to approach the patient and decided that it would be best to start by caring for her basic biological needs and improving her comfort. This kind of "mothering," in which the patient is cared for on the simplest level, may be of great importance in initiating a relationship with a withdrawn patient.

January 8

Miss Harris: I told her we thought her nails were too long and that we have to take care of her, so we were going to cut them. I went in there with two other nurses, prepared to hold her if necessary. We had to take her arms and then she let us cut them. She was much more responsive after we cut her nails. Then I suggested that she take a bath. At first she refused, but she finally did.

SOCIOLOGIST: In other words, you started at the most elementary level. The first indication you give a patient that you really care is by taking care of her most elementary needs.

MISS HARRIS: Yes, and if she doesn't eat, I spoon-feed her. But if she wants to eat by herself, I let her eat.

SOCIOLOGIST: I can imagine how horrible she must feel if nobody takes care of her for even these elementary things. I think patients want you to care about them and want you to take care of them. When she can't bathe or eat it would be well to watch carefully what she does and how she reacts to you. Whatever plan you work out to get her to bathe or eat, be prepared to change it. If you've started her in the bath and she gives you the cue that she'll do it herself, let her do it.

Another way in which the nurse decided to approach Miss Levin initially was to see her for short periods only. She was asked her reasons for this.

January 10

MISS HARRIS: With some withdrawn patients like Miss Levin I might go many days without having a successful contact. Then if I'm not getting any satisfaction from spending so much time with her, I get discouraged. Maybe she can't take a sustained contact at this time. Maybe it's better to have brief contacts that last only a few minutes but are frequent throughout the day. If you add them up it could be quite a lot, and be very useful to her. These small contacts made when I bring her some milk, fix her bed, offer her some gum or candy—the little extra things—might be very meaningful to her.

After a short period, Miss Harris was able to move from brief contacts to more sustained relations with Miss Levin. She recognized the importance of waiting and giving the patient the time she needed to respond.

January 17

MISS HARRIS: Unless you have fifteen minutes to sit down with her when you ask her a question, you don't get an answer. Some personnel go in there and ask her a question and get no response. They don't wait. When I ask her to do something I don't push her but wait as long as necessary for a reply.

SOCIOLOGIST: Have you ever tried to put yourself in the patient's place and figure out what she's feeling or what she thinks about you in these situations?

MISS HARRIS: I've tried, but it's awfully hard. Sometimes I think she thinks I'm just pestering her or trying to push her into a kind of behavior she doesn't want. Sometimes I think she enjoys being with me.

Frequently, in the development of a relationship with a withdrawn patient, the patient becomes verbally hostile to the nurse or attacks her physically. Miss Harris was asked how she handled Miss Levin on such occasions.

January 19

MISS HARRIS: I don't feel that her hostility is really directed at me, although she does direct it toward me. She has a deep-rooted belief that everybody is trying to coerce her into doing things, and she thinks I'm also trying to do this. Maybe if I accept the fact that she puts me in a position of authority and feels I'm trying to coerce her, she can work it out on me and she might get over her anger and the feeling that everybody is forcing her to do things. Also, I think it's better for her to express this hostility than to be so passive and withdrawn. I feel if I can handle the attack and stick with her, it might be an important step in bringing her out of her withdrawal.

In addition to hostility, the nurse had to sustain various forms of rejection and rebuff from the patient during the course of their relationship.

January 23

SOCIOLOGIST: Why do you continue to work with her and go back every morning even though she keeps rebuffing you? I remember you were very much disappointed that first morning.

MISS HARRIS: I don't know. I feel that I get some response from her now, even though at first she wouldn't talk and wouldn't get up or do anything. At first when I tried to talk with her, she told me that a person who is very sick doesn't feel like talking. Later on I asked her to play dominoes, and she did. She also listened while I read to her.

SOCIOLOGIST: Are you saying that even though she rebuffs you now, you had little successes with her before and you feel you can repeat these—that when she chases you away and is sarcastic you can keep at the back of your mind that you were able to get a good response once and it can happen again?

MISS HARRIS: Yes. The other thing is that I'm interested in her and curious to see what happens. I want to know what she's going to do when I go in and talk to her or when I ask her to go for a walk with me.

The nurse met more rejection and withdrawal, but persisted nevertheless.

January 28

MISS HARRIS: The other day when I came into her room she said, "Get out right now." It threw me. She was very hostile, and mimicked me. So I just stood there. She kept it up and I finally walked out. After a while I took her tray in and she was a little friendlier. I invited her to the picnic and said I'd like to take her, but she wouldn't go. I came back and asked her again. This time I didn't get any answer.

SOCIOLOGIST: She's really giving you the silent treatment.

MISS HARRIS: She's just shutting me out completely. But I don't think it will last, and I've become very much interested in trying to find out what's happening. The other day when I asked her if she wanted me to come back to see her, she said, "I don't know." I said, "If you don't know, I'll just come back to see you anyway, because I want to see you." When I came back she didn't say hello to me, she didn't even look at me. I stayed with her for about fifteen minutes in silence.

The nurse explored the ups and downs of her relations with the patient and began to understand herself and the patient a little better.

February 4

MISS HARRIS: I wanted to take Miss Levin for a walk. I suggested this to her and got no response. So I said, "You think about it and I'll ask you again." I asked later in the day, and she still didn't respond. I asked her again the next day. Well, she had thought about it and she agreed to go. I didn't put any pressure on her, just gave her time to make up her mind. I also think it's important to give her a choice. One of the big dangers with withdrawn patients like her is to think she's so ill that she's not able to make any choices. She can about some things and not about others, and we have to figure out what these things are.

SOCIOLOGIST: I think it was important that you were willing to wait. This was the first time she's been out of bed for quite a while.

MISS HARRIS: Yes. I took her for the walk and we did some other things together this past week, but now she's gone back to rejecting me. She's been pushing me away.

SOCIOLOGIST: How is she pushing you away?

MISS HARRIS: When I come in she won't get up, nor will she comb her hair. She thinks that I'll just go away and leave her alone. She asks me to go away.

SOCIOLOGIST: What do you do?

MISS HARRIS: Once I just stayed with her for a little while. Yesterday I was much annoyed. She said, "I can't understand why you keep coming back when you know I want to be alone." She also said, "You know I'm not well enough to get up and walk." I was so annoyed.

SOCIOLOGIST: What were you annoyed at?

MISS HARRIS: It was really because she didn't meet my own expectations, I suppose.

SOCIOLOGIST: You felt that she could get up, that she had before. It seems that you have to keep two things in mind at the same time. On the one hand, you accept the fact that she feels she can't get up and walk. This is her feeling and you respect it. But you also know she's capable of more than that, even though she can't do it right now. You're willing to wait for the time when she can. So it seems that she both can and can't get up and walk.

MISS HARRIS: I just got impatient with her.

SOCIOLOGIST: You have to become aware of your annoyance and also not feel guilty about it. In the same way that you accept her problems and difficulties, you have to accept your own reactions of anger and guilt.

MISS HARRIS: I wonder if you could give me any ideas about how to handle her rejection of me.

SOCIOLOGIST: It seems to me you have to depend on your feelings. When she says, "I don't want to see you," does she really mean it, or not? You might even say to her that you can't decide whether she really wants you to leave. Then see what she does. Watch her. Don't only listen to her words, see how she moves. Does she move away or does she move forward? Does she frown? Pick up any cue you can to tell you how she really feels. If you decide to leave her, tell her you'll come back, and do so.

Miss Harris: Going back is really important. Yesterday I sensed that maybe she was wondering if I was coming back. I did go back for a few minutes.

Sociologist: Its importance is in the fact that you tell her your relationship goes on even though you had a difficult and annnoying time yesterday; that doesn't destroy the good feeling you had.

Miss Harris: If she knows that she can be hostile toward me and that I accept this by going back, maybe she'll get rid of some of these feelings. Maybe she will feel more secure with me.

Sociologist: Maybe she'll learn that you can have both hostile and friendly feelings toward the same person, and the hostile ones don't destroy the friendly ones. It's important to build up a basic feeling of confidence and trust that the relationship will go on no matter what. The patient is afraid things will always come to a bad end. Taking the hostility and coming back builds up the opposite of that. What else happens between you and her?

Miss Harris: Sometimes I just sit there silently. I've learned to do this, and it's part of our being together.

Sociologist: What do you do when you're silent?

Miss Harris: I think of what's going on. What does she think about me? What's going on between us? What am I thinking about her? I try to study the situation, how I feel and what the patient is thinking. Another thing she has taught me is how to be silent.

Sociologist: It's not easy to be silent when you're in a room with a patient. Have you noticed that there's more than one type of silence?

Miss Harris: Silence is a fascinating thing. Sometimes when you interrupt a silence you can create disorder.

Sociologist: Do you mean that silence is an activity, and when you interrupt it you start another activity going?

Miss Harris: Yes. Silences aren't all hostile.

Sociologist: I think silence can range from one extreme of sullen hostility to the other extreme of real sympathy and understanding.

Miss Harris: I've experienced both of these with Miss Levin. She also shows a thoughtful silence, when she seems to be trying to work something out.

Sociologist: Then there's a silence in which the two people are in each other's presence, accept this, and feel comfortable about it, and receive some support from each other.

Miss Harris: To observe these different silences is fascinating and is part of my becoming more aware of what is happening between me and the patient.

Sociologist: Could you give me some examples of this increased awareness?

Miss Harris: Something that made me sit up and take notice was recognizing that some of my so-called good intentions for patients are really wishes for my own satisfaction or in order to meet my own standards. When you get to looking at these things you wonder. . . .

Sociologist: As a nurse you're supposed to be selfless, devoting yourself to the needs of the other. But the nurse also has needs, and if she discovers that and takes her own needs also into account, it will probably be easier to take care of patients' needs.

Miss Harris: Sure. When I ask a patient to go out on the porch with me because it's so hot in her room, I'm also asking for myself because I'm hot.

Miss Harris continued to have her ups and downs with the patient. Sometimes Miss Levin accepted her, and the nurse took her for walks and carried on extensive conversations with her. At other times the patient returned to her silent, rejecting, behavior. When Miss Levin was in one of the latter states, the nurse was asked to review her relationship with the patient and try to evaluate it.

February 20

Sociologist: I'm interested in why you selected Miss Levin as someone you were interested in, when she was so withdrawn.

Miss Harris: I felt that she would accept me, and when I sat with her and she let me stay I felt passive acceptance from her. Also, I felt a lot of hopefulness about her—that there was something to work with in her.

Sociologist: What was it that indicated the hopefulness?

Miss Harris: It seemed that I got some response from her the first day I sat with her, and that was hopeful for a relationship. Then I began picking up clues that indicated a progressive response. I could get her out on the porch; then she went for a walk with me. One time she asked me to bring her a magazine. When I brought it, she was really interested.

Sociologist: In our last talk you were somewhat discouraged about her renewed withdrawal after you had had so many good contacts with her. What's happened?

Miss Harris: She still stays in bed, though I can get her to the shower. But she hasn't been hostile toward me this week.

Sociologist: You seem to be pretty persistent—even though she pushes you away, you go back.

Miss Harris: I want our relationship to continue. I know she doesn't dislike me.

SOCIOLOGIST: You seem to have a quiet determination to continue, as if to say, "I'm going to continue our relationship because I feel strongly enough about it and I feel strongly enough about you."

MISS HARRIS: Another reason I continue is because she teaches me a lot. I've become more observant about myself. Also, she teaches me things about her. When she gets quite close to me she soon has to withdraw and push me away. I've learned that she thinks everyone is against her. She feels unworthy, and that she's against herself, and that she doesn't like herself. She actually tells me these things. I've also learned to be patient with her. I wait until she responds to me, and I notice when she responds and what cues she gives me.

SOCIOLOGIST: In this way, waiting wasn't something you had to struggle with. It was easier to wait patiently when you were interested in observing yourself and the patient. And, when you waited for her response, you were respectful of the patient's need to go at her own pace.

We can now summarize some of the chief characteristics of the problem situation in which a patient is withdrawn and some of the personnel responses that are helpful in reducing patient withdrawal. We have said previously that the first step is to become aware of the patient's withdrawal. This awareness often means that the nurse sees the patient differently. When his withdrawal is not noticed, she experiences him as an inert, undifferentiated mass, without being able to specify much in a concrete way about his activities or personality. Or she experiences vague discomfort in herself that tends to prevent her from seeing the patient. When she becomes aware of the patient as a withdrawn person who needs help, the patient becomes more alive and real and she notices more details of his activities. The nurse can now observe many subtleties about the patient's behavior. He makes an impression on her; she recognizes his effect upon her as well as her effect upon him. The patient begins to count; he becomes a source of concern, interest, curiosity, sympathy, identification, and difficulty.

When the nurse has focused her attention on a withdrawn patient she must then call upon her patience and persistence. The patient can "wear her down." One day she will feel she is making headway with him, and the next day she will feel she is getting nowhere. The patient may need to find out if the nurse really cares and if her interest in him is sincere. If he is convinced of this, he may be friendly and active with her, but this friendliness may change suddenly. The nurse must expect these variations and in some way accept them as part of the process of bringing the patient into more satisfying relations with others. She must be clear about her own expectations and how they get in her way or help her with the patient. If she expects uninterrupted progress, rapid change, or that the patient will be easy to deal with, she is likely to become discouraged and easily give up. If the nurse has a specific preestablished goal and feels that the patient ought to reach it in a specified time, she may be disappointed. The patient may not fulfill the nurse's expectations, and the nurse, therefore, may develop feelings of failure and withdraw her interest from him.

It is important for the nurse to recognize that the withdrawn patient may try her patience, strain her resources, make her feel angry, hopeless, helpless, and weary. It is also important for her to expect temporary failures and realize that it may take a long time to see a change in the patient. If she can look upon each difficult incident as something the patient has to do before he can trust her, as something to be curious about, as something challenging that can be understood, and as something potentially rich in learning experience for her, then she may not have to give up. If she learns how to observe the patient carefully and con-sistently, she may find these difficult incidents easier to cope with. We cannot give the nurse a formula for developing patience and persistence. These qualities need to evolve for each nurse in her own situation, as she tries to recognize the processes that interfere with their development and as she tries to use her ingenuity and imagination in changing her behavior as the situation and the patient require.

In order to discover the activity that fits at a particular time, the nurse must be alert to the signs the patient gives; she must be curious, grope for, and seek these cues. Each situation contains its own challenge as to what the patient will accept and respond to and which type of activity from the nurse will stimulate him to participate or will mobilize his responsiveness. The nurse often cannot tell in advance what will work with the patient and must try to go along with him or stick close to him, using all her sensitivity to tune herself in on the patient. Much of what she does may be on the basis of hunch, intuition, or guess. But she can watch her effect on the patient, to see how he responds and whether his participation increases or appears to be more satisfying to him. With repeated experiences the nurse may come to rely on her feelings and her intuitive responses to the patient. She may also learn why some of her responses to the patient were effective and thus be able to develop more reliable and more consistently effective activity in the future. This, of course, involves a constant searching for alternative ways of trying to reach the patient, noticing his response to the alternative chosen, and adjusting on the basis of his response. In developing an appropriate response, the nurse must keep alert to her own feelings as they are aroused in the situation but not focus on these exclusively. She must keep her primary focus on the patient and use her feelings as clues to what is happening to him. She must be able to distinguish between situations in which the patient *has to* be withdrawn and those in which he will participate with her if her approach is appropriate and sensitive.

The nurse is not alone in her attempts to bring withdrawn patients into greater participation. Her efforts take place in a group, and the nursing staff as a group can work out ways of helping a particular nurse. The questions that have to be asked are: How can personnel organize themselves so that patients are not overlooked? How can the staff develop the attitude that the withdrawn patients' participation or lack of it is a problem to be constantly considered? How can the initiative and enthusiasm of nurses be mobilized so that they use imagination in devising ways of approaching the patient? What are useful ways in which nurses can give support and encouragement to each other in dealing with withdrawn patients?

« 5 »

The Patient Is Hallucinating,
Delusional, or Self-Preoccupied

TO some extent each person has his own private inner world,
meaningful to him alone. At the same time he has the capacity to understand others and to share experiences with them.
Others, in turn, are able to understand him. One says a person is
mentally ill if his private world dominates his relations with
others, if his ideas are distorted and indicate that he has lost his
grasp on reality, if others cannot understand him and he cannot
understand them most of the time, if his detachment and isolation
become extreme, or if he engages in actions that are atypical and
strange. More specifically, we say this person is hallucinating,
delusional, deeply preoccupied (probably with inner voices or
fantastic thoughts), or manneristic and stereotyped in his gestures. In this book this kind of behavior is called *autistic behavior*.
By this term we mean actions, thoughts, feelings, ideas, and experiences that are highly private, inappropriate, distorted, and not
easily understood by other people. Nursing personnel are familiar
with the ways in which autistic behavior may be expressed: The
patient hears voices giving him directions that no one else hears;
he feels he is being tortured and persecuted by sparks coming
from electric wires; he believes he must not get close to other
people because poison gas is coming out of their mouths; he
thinks there is an opening in his head and that other people can
read his mind; he raves, rants, and threatens to destroy the
world; he laughs or cries at times when there seems no reason to
do so; he sits and stares with a vacant look in his eyes and seems
to be "out of this world"; he talks in a confused way that is im-

possible to understand; he moves his hand in a circular pattern over and over; or he strikes a pose and holds it for long periods of time.

We will try to develop some understanding of what is involved in situations in which the patient responds with autistic behavior. Illustrations will be given of ways of dealing with autistic patients that we have found useful. Nursing personnel can best use the experiences we present by translating and adapting them for each autistic patient in their care.

One error nurses might make about autistic patients is to think that they are completely unaware of what is going on around them. This interpretation is made especially of patients who are deeply preoccupied or who seem to be off in the clouds. A patient may frequently be concentrating so hard on his own fantasies and thoughts that he appears oblivious to his environment, but we believe that in most instances the patient has some awareness of his environment, even if this awareness is only peripheral and not very clear to him. It seems to us that most of the time he is paying close attention to what is going on around him but does not show his awareness. In some instances we have found that many weeks after an event has occurred the patient can recall what happened in a situation to which he seemed oblivious at the time. Thus, it seems unwise for the nurse to discount the autistic patient's sensitivity and awareness.

However, it should be made clear that the patient's recognition and awareness of an event does not mean that he necessarily sees it the same way the nurse does. As a matter of fact, he often sees it very differently. But the fact of his *seeing it* is important. Once the nurse accepts the idea that the patient hears, sees, and experiences the events around him—even though he may distort their meaning or not see them as they actually happen—she will no longer act as if her words and actions do not affect the patient. She will avoid such disrespectful behavior as talking about him in his presence, as if he were not there. She will recognize that even though the patient appears remote, detached, and unaffected by events, *she and others are having some influence on him.*

No matter how distorted or twisted a patient's perceptions or interpretations are, they are not totally so. We might say that the patient *distorts selected aspects* of the environment. How widespread such distortion is—how much is distorted and how much is realistic—the nurse can try to determine for each patient. In inquiring into this matter she may discover that in some areas of his relations with others and about some subjects the patient is quite realistic. In other areas he is on and off, sometimes realistic in his appraisal and sometimes quite distorted. In still other areas he may be misinterpreting his environment all the time. In those areas in which he is severely handicapped, maintaining delusions and hallucinations in their grossest and most obvious form, the nurse can ask herself how firmly and strongly these distortions are held and consider the possible ways of making some inroad into the false beliefs or imaginary occurrences, even if only temporarily. In those areas where the patient vacillates in his autistic behavior, the nurse might be able to identify the situations in which he is more realistic and those that bring about his autistic behavior. If she has some awareness of the ways in which and the circumstances under which the patient perceives his environment with distortion, she may be able to find ways of relating to him so that his distortions become less extensive and compelling and interfere less in his relations with others.

How the nurse reacts to the patient in these situations is also important. She may become annoyed with his incomprehensible behavior and become restrictive of him. If she becomes angry, she may insist that the patient "stop it," or she may feel that "he ought to act differently." She may be extremely surprised at the patient's fantastic thoughts or his misinterpretations. Confused by his talk, she may throw up her hands in despair and think, "If he's as crazy as that, he'll never get well." She may expect the patient to continue his autistic behavior because "that's the way he is." If she is seldom able to understand him, the nurse may become indifferent and dismiss his behavior by calling it "that crazy stuff." Because she cannot tell how they get started, continue, and stop, the patient's autistic activities may discourage her and lead her to avoid or reject him. When she experiences some of the feeling underlying the patient's autistic behavior, she may become anxious and, forgetting about the patient, think of ways she can make herself more comfortable. By becoming aware of these attitudes and feelings and her consequent actions, the nurse might remove some of the blocks that stand in the way of her helping the patient become more realistic, more concrete, more "down-to-earth."

It is inevitable that these patients will misinterpret some of the nurse's actions. If she is surprised or disappointed by this, or if she feels that the patient is unfair or ungrateful, these feelings are likely to get in her way. However, if she expects that autistic behavior will occur and if she is able to accept it, it may be easier for her to understand it and to help the patient change it. In order to show what is involved in situations where patients behave autistically and how nurses respond to this behavior, we will focus first on patients' autistic talk, then on patients' misinterpretations, and, finally, on patients' preoccupation with themselves.

Autistic Communication

It is important for the nurse to recognize that *the patient's autistic talk is meaningful to him*. It is *his way* of expressing himself and approaching others. By paying close attention, the nurse may be able to get a clue to the meaning of the patient's communication: what he is trying to say, how he feels, what he wants, or what needs he is trying to have fulfilled. Any exchange in which the patient feels he is understood is useful for him. But accepting the patient's autistic talk *by listening to him*, and thereby accepting him, is just as important as understanding the meaning or significance of the talk itself. Even if the nurse cannot understand the meaning of the patient's statements, giving him the opportunity to talk and accepting his way of relating with her are helpful to him.

Sometimes a patient's communication is so elusive that the nurse has only a momentary, faint glimmer of what he is driving at, but immediately afterward she is in the dark again. In the following example the patient writes:

> I dreamed of a tree and the many bodies dumped in the branches saying prayers for their blessings. I dreamed every human alive

walked in a procession two by two, men on the left, women on the right around the globe; their eyes sparkled like diamonds. Their lips were faithful to their love for the hours of knowing all answers. The leaves turned into emeralds. The sky was of a mosaic turquoise and sapphire. The moon was a moonstone. The sun was a golden ball. The clouds were pearls. Home is the heart. Robin's-egg blue, orange shadow, the eyes. The free world cried for salvation, for their skin. I'll see you in Hell. Every human is crazy. I have been in the room of the damned. I will tell you about it. There was no sense, there was no understanding. There was no fair play. There was no hope. There was no obedience. The men were transformed into walking white flames. The women were changed into glittering fairy queens. Ivory faces, ivory arms, ivory hands, ivory legs, ivory feet, ebony hair— moss agate grass, grieving dust. This is the realization; there is no going back. This is the land of no return. With a trowel buried and spaded away. Into the tunnel into fairyland, which existed under the grass. Fairies were busy at work making silver shoes, silver slippers, silver tones, silver skirts, silver dresses, silver chairs, silver earrings, silver boats, silver cars, silver tables, silver rugs, silver wall paper, silver everything, silver money, silver brains. One fairy was manufacturing character, he took a glass of pride and a grain of good fun and a grain of independence and squeezed them together. My beloved is breathing, my beloved is grave. Humans are shadows of their creator. They are transitory. We are bad ships that never reach port. Wisdom is their desire. Silence makes a well person, questions make a sick person. Ask and it is not given, seek and you will not find it. Quiet rest. Health is not bought. Health is an inward relationship in which the other person thinks and feels. Health is the normal, being well is the common heritage. A well person does not get bothered, does not get nervous. A well person is composed. A well person does not complain. A well person does not tear up clothes. A well person does not break things. A well person does not swear. A well person does not sin. A well person is polite. A well person is not influenced by other people. Monday I am in here to get well. I am in here to get it straight in my own mind. How to prevent another hospitalization. I think that I should have a private detective to prevent a man or woman from dragging me in here against my will. Asking for the door to be opened has gotten me no place. I feel as though I am having a nervous breakdown and I don't want to admit it. Experience has proven that cigarettes have not gotten me well. When I leave the hospital, I'm going to take to drinking. I have no evidence that contact with another human being is helpful. I want to investigate this from the beginning. Before this, I have always shrunk from human contact.

Despite its vagueness the nurses felt they understood something of what she was trying to communicate. One nurse interpreted it in the following way:

> The patient was groping for some clarity about her situation, trying to see through it. In the course of this groping, she escapes into fantasy where the world is pretty and her situation is happy; then she goes to the other extreme, feeling despair and hopelessness. In addition, she becomes puzzled and doubting about the way things are, produces some delusional ideas about her situation, and then indicates that she has a slight realistic grasp on her situation. Throughout she seems to be asking for help for her difficulties and discomfort.

Another nurse, in discussing the patient with a colleague, gave her interpretation of the patient's autistic communication:

> I have the feeling that Joan is telling us something about the relations she has had in the past and about the kinds of relations she would like to have. She says the world is beautiful, but that there is something wrong with the people in it. Everybody has a need to love and to be loved, but people just talk about it and don't actually do it. [Their lips are faithful. People go in pairs, but they go in a procession.] People keep a lot of distance between them. One of the ways they do this is to associate with a lot of people and not develop any understanding or intimacy with individual persons. [No sense, no understanding, no fair play.] She feels that it is horrible the way people [she] live[s], with no warmth or tenderness. [The room of the damned. No hope.] Even though it is horrible, she can't change the past [there is no going back], and she despairs that people have [she has] to live this way.
>
> At this point it seems that the patient becomes more anxious and retreats into a fairyland. In her imagination she can arrange the world in the way she would like to have it—beautiful, bright, and shining.
>
> She talks again about people and their relations with each other. They want to understand each other, and how to live together happily, but they never find out how to meet their needs, and they don't know how to find out. Then she gets a little closer to herself and talks about mental health. [A well person.] She uses the term "I," and this is a hopeful sign. She seems to be a little more comfortable and ready to deal with her own life situation and the problems in it. [I'm here to get things straight.] She thinks that life outside the hospital might be possible for her, but that she may not know how to manage it.

[When I leave the hospital.] She also wants to find out how she got to be the way she is. [I want to investigate this from the beginning.] She ends up by showing that she has more hope for forming a meaningful relation with others. [Before this I have always shrunk from human contact.]

The foregoing examples illustrate the interpretations a nurse might make of a patient's autistic communication. She can react in a number of ways in trying to understand it. To mention only a few: She may have a vague intimation of what the patient is driving at and grope for a response to that part of his talk she can grasp. She might try to detect the feeling tone that accompanies the patient's talk and in this way determine something of his meaning. She might interpret (to herself or to the patient) the meaning of the patient's words, guessing at the allusions he is making, and act in accordance with her interpretation. By showing her puzzlement about his unclear statements, she can try to help the patient clarify his meaning and get him to help her understand what he is trying to say. She can listen intently and show that she is interested in hearing what the patient is saying, even though its meaning may not be clear to her. She may have to listen to many words that are not understandable before she sees some meaning in his talk. In responding to the patient, the nurse can be careful not to reinforce his vagueness by giving him similarly vague, indefinite, and obscure replies.

In situations where the nurse selects certain aspects of the patient's talk to respond to, it is important for her to notice the effects of her responses. In the example below the nurse observes the patient's reactions to her comments and changes her behavior on the basis of these reactions.

MISS ALLEN: She kept talking about the same things she usually does. She said, "I'm sick and nobody cares what happens to me." And then some stuff about, "I don't know anything about the price of eggs." Then there was a lot about, "I just sit on the toilet and blood runs all over the place." She stayed on blood awhile and then she went from there to a lot of names of people I don't know. Then she started singing, the same repetitive tune—"Give My Regards to Broadway." We finally got her dressed and went out in the hall and she was still talking. She sat in a rocking chair and I sat on the arm.

I said, "It's good to be able to talk to you and hear what you have to say; we're really interested." She shut right up, and I thought maybe I shouldn't have said it. I kept quiet and then she said, "Nobody understands." I said, "We try to understand. We understand some of the time." She kept on saying she's impossible and I said, "We don't feel that you're impossible." This seemed to quiet her down a little.

During one conversation the patient may vary from realistic talk to autistic talk. How the nurse reacts to and accepts this variation may have an important effect on the patient's continuing autistic behavior.

MISS BARKER: At first she talked about the meeting and I could understand that, and then she went off about encrusted brains and psychoanalysis and crud. I said, "I'm trying hard to understand you but I can't." She said, "It's even harder when you don't understand." I said, "That's a profound statement." Then she went on about "Self-integration is equal to self-engulfment." I said, "Do you mean self-involvement?" She said, "Now you're on the ball." I still didn't know what she was talking about. There was so much that I just couldn't follow. But some of it I could understand. She asked me where I went to school. I told her, and she told me where she went to school. Sometimes I'd get some straight conversations; most of the time she'd go wandering off. When she talked about Shakespeare, religion, history, and the universal truth I would tell her I couldn't follow her. I just felt pretty inadequate and stupid not being able to follow her.

Sometimes the nurse can grasp the significance of part of what the patient is saying and is able to carry on a partially realistic conversation with him. She may be able to develop the patient's seemingly irrational comments into a rational conversation between them. It is out of such communication that the nurse and patient develop meaningful exchange and some understanding of each other.

MRS. BELL: When I went into the patient's room she wanted to know what was going on and then she'd go way off into something that I couldn't understand. She said everybody was looking at her, and she went on about Ducky-Lucky when the sky fell. Then it rang a bell, and I said, "Oh, that's the story of Chicken Little."
SOCIOLOGIST: Which story?

MRS. BELL: The one where a little chicken starts running because an acorn hit him on the head and he thinks the sky is falling and the world is coming to an end. Anyway we sat down and went through this story, and after that she was in pretty good shape.

SOCIOLOGIST: What do you think went on?

MRS. BELL: She was sitting there with this silly giggle and faraway look, saying, "Ducky-Lucky, a piece of sky has hit me on the head."

SOCIOLOGIST: Why do you think you were able to get her to talk in a fairly realistic way?

MRS. BELL: We retraced the story and found out what she was thinking about.

SOCIOLOGIST: In effect you told her, "You're not so crazy. I can understand you. I can talk with you about it, and we know what we're talking about."

In some situations the nurse may try to follow through on the patient's ideas by asking him to clarify them. By bringing her questions into the conversation the nurse might show the patient her interest in understanding him, and also by interjecting her comments she might for a short time bring the patient into a more realistic relation with her.

MISS ALLEN: When I asked her what her sigh meant, she said, "It means understanding." She said, "Yeah, that's what it means, understanding." And I said, "Understanding of what?" "Well," she said, "You know, when everything's been so sort of messed up and all is piled in one big heap and then you get some understanding, why it's sort of like a revelation to you." So then I said, "Understanding about what? Is it about yourself?" "Oh no," she said, "not always." She said, "I think if you wanted to call it something you could call it universal insight." So then she really started giving this terrific lot of psychotic stuff which I started breaking into. She said, "Well, it goes clear back to culture and to culturation and a bunch of stuff that people dream up and base their lives on." And she said, "If you want to take geographic areas, there isn't one single one that you can't find a terrible mess in, that people have built their lives on and think they're right." And then she got way off, and I said, "I'm not following you at all." I said, "You were talking about universal insight and we were talking about your sighing, and now you're talking about history and geography." "Well," she said, "It's all a big mess. Everything that has gone into it." She got way off the beam on that and I couldn't get her back. And finally she said, "Well, isn't it enough to tell you that it's universal insight?" And I said, "Well, I don't under-

stand this, but you don't need to talk about it if you don't want to."
She was saying—I wish I could remember all that she said—but I do
recall her saying, "There's a big mess up here," and she was describing it geographically—"And then down behind there's another
whirlpool, and up in front there. . . ." And pretty soon I had a
visual image of anatomy, and thought that she wasn't describing
geography, but was talking about her body. But I just thought, "My
gosh, what is she getting at?" And I listened very hard. She was talking very fast, and if anybody had come in, I'm sure he would have
thought she was completely off the beam, although at the slightest
minute I could bring her right back and stop it. When I asked,
"Now wait, what did you say?" she'd repeat it.

Sometimes the nurse-patient relationship is sufficiently good
and the patient is in "good enough shape" to be able to explain
her obscure or elusive communication to the nurse.

MISS ALLEN: She wrote two poems and she wanted to see what I
thought of them. In the first one the world is all women, never any
men. One line was, "Never any men, but sometimes even men," and
the last line was "Fourteen." The other poem was called "Suspended
City." The poem was all one line. "And the mistakes of the world are
fallen into the gray muck below." That was the second poem. And
then she started telling me that her entire personality was around
these two poems. So she went on and on. Some of it made pretty good
sense and some didn't. The second meant that the world would never
get to the place where we could actually live together. And so there
would finally be such turmoil and strife that the cities would bounce
off the earth and be suspended in air, and the mistakes we made
would fall down into the gray muck of the earth. That was what the
second poem meant. The first poem meant that in her life there are
never any men. But if this were true all over, that there were just
women, then the world wouldn't go on. So in order to make it even
there were men; that was what the "even" was, so the world would go
on. The "fourteen" has to do with the fourteen patients on the ward.

At times the nurse can be helpful to a patient without understanding his specific reference. Something goes on between nurse
and patient on a nonverbal, emotional level, which is difficult to
identify but is, nevertheless, useful for the patient.

MRS. GILBERT: Beatrice kept pleading with me to get her a brain
operation. At first I said, "Beatrice, it won't help you." She just began to cry and plead. I rubbed her leg, which had a cramp in it,

and she settled down. But she started asking again for the operation. I said, "Beatrice, I wouldn't want anyone I was fond of to have a brain operation."

SOCIOLOGIST: Did you try to find out what's behind her statement, what it means?

MRS. GILBERT: I did say, "I think you're asking for something desperately, and I wonder what it is. I wish I knew."

SOCIOLOGIST: In this way you tell her that you understand that she wants something that she isn't getting. The best you may be able to do is to let her know that you recognize that she's suffering a lot and that you'll stay with her and try to help as much as you can.

MRS. GILBERT: I started feeling desperate myself. I wanted to do something to relieve her.

SOCIOLOGIST: It's difficult to accept the fact that being there with her is doing something?

MRS. GILBERT: Well, I just sat there with her and she calmed down.

SOCIOLOGIST: It's hard to accept the idea that maybe that's all you can do right now. You have the feeling that you should do more, or that if you could only say the right thing it would help her. Do you know what "more" you would like to do?

MRS. GILBERT: I don't think I know.

SOCIOLOGIST: I think the patient doesn't really know what she's asking for, and neither do you know what you're expected to give or what you expect yourself to give. You feel dissatisfaction in what you are giving and she feels dissatisfied in what she's getting. The more you become aware of what's involved in this situation, the greater the possibility will be of your being of some use to her. But you have already been helpful by trying to understand, by sitting with her, and by doing the many little things with her that you've done.

A few days later the nurse again talks about this patient.

MRS. GILBERT: I think Beatrice is getting to the point where she doesn't have to keep asking me for something like a brain operation so that I will stay with her. I went back to her after we talked and said, "Maybe we don't mean the same thing by this [the brain operation]. Can you tell me what you mean?" She didn't answer but became relaxed and quieted down. I get the feeling now when she asks for it that I don't have to interpret her request and that she doesn't expect me to give her an answer.

In addition to responding verbally to the patient's autistic talk, doing something for the patient sometimes helps. Offering him some food, taking him for a walk, rubbing his back, and the like, might help him focus on something real and concrete through which the nurse and patient can relate to each other in a mutually understandable way. In some situations, the patient might understand simple relations on an elementary level, such as physical contact, and be able to respond to these when he is not able to respond to the nurse's words. Often nonverbal responses—the nurse's body movements, her approach and general attitude—can be meaningful and reassuring to the autistic patient.

MISINTERPRETATIONS OF THE ENVIRONMENT

How can the nurse understand and handle the patient's misinterpretations of the environment, his false beliefs or perceptions? Usually it is very difficult to learn directly from the patient the meaning of or the reasons for his peculiar or obscure behavior. Ordinarily, he is too suspicious of others or too secretive about his private thoughts to reveal them readily to anyone else. Once in a while, if he knows the nurse quite well and has had good experiences with her in the past, he might tell her about them.

> MISS HOWELL: Yesterday I said to him, "John, I want to ask you a question. Would you answer it?" I thought I'd go at it that way and see what his mood was, whether it was suspicious or not. He said, "Sure, go ahead." I said, "Why do you wear that coat all the time, day in and day out? It's full of holes and isn't very clean." He said, "So I can have some privacy around here." I asked, "How does this give you privacy?" He said, "I didn't ask to be brought here. I wasn't asked if I wanted to associate with the patients or personnel. By keeping this coat on it means I'm not here." I said, "Do you mean something like a magic cloak?" He said, "That's right." I said, "Are you also trying to say that by keeping your coat on it means that you're not going to expose yourself to these other people, to let them see what you're like?" Again he said, "That's right."
>
> He also told me that the nurses are plotting to murder him here. He said his mother's a bitch and just hates him. The nurses are in cahoots with the mother. All I said was that I knew the nurses and I knew they weren't planning to murder him. I didn't argue with him; I just told him I didn't agree with him.

In the foregoing illustration the patient could reveal his distortions to the nurse. The nurse, in turn, could comfortably disagree with the patient. Because of their good relationship, the patient was also able to tell the nurse why he had to attack other people. He said, "As soon as I get close to anybody I feel that I destroy them. That's why I have to keep driving people away; in order to preserve them I have to attack them." By this statement the patient indicated in an indirect way the reason he had to maintain the idea that others were trying to hurt him. Because the patient was afraid that his friendliness with others would destroy them, he had to find a way of prohibiting this friendliness. One way to do this is by attacking others. But he must have some "reason" for such attacks. The patient finds the reason quite unconsciously by imagining that others are trying to destroy him. In order to save himself he attacks them first. In this unconscious way he saves the personnel from destruction by him.

One of the things a nurse can do in dealing with a patient's misinterpretations—his delusions or hallucinations—is to deny that they are real, or to disagree with them. However, in so doing the nurse must first be sure that the patient's statements are in fact delusional. Without realizing it, a nurse may assume that because a patient has been delusional and has hallucinated in the past he is necessarily similarly delusional or hallucinating in a particular situation or is distorting reality all the time. It is easy to label the patient "delusional" and by attaching this label to him, dismiss the possibility of his "making sense" and being realistic in some situations. The patient might have his autistic behavior reinforced considerably by the nurse's consistent and invariable attitude that he is "just a crazy delusional patient." In order to avoid this, the nurse must be careful to validate the nature of the real situation or the falsity of the patient's beliefs before she makes an unequivocal evaluation that the patient is hallucinating or delusional. In some situations the delusion is obvious and easily validated; in others it is not so simple to establish reality. In the example that follows an aide makes a number of attempts to determine the facts before she decides that the patient is distorting reality.

A patient was drinking coffee at lunch time. He complained to the aide that the cream was sour. She took the cream from him, went into the kitchen and poured him some cream from a bottle that was already open. On tasting this cream the patient again complained that it was sour. The aide went back to the kitchen and asked the dietician to open a bottle of the freshest cream available. She brought this cream to the patient and tasted it herself. Again the patient said the cream was sour. The aide told him that this was fresh cream, the best they had. She also said, "It tastes sour to you, but I drank some of it in the kitchen and it tasted all right to me." The patient finished drinking his coffee without any cream in it.

The aide did not assume that the patient was delusional, nor did she assume that he was accurate. Nor did she ignore him. She tried to find out what was reality in this situation. When her checking convinced her that the difficulty lay in the patient's taste, she could then disagree with him and point out how she saw the situation.

It is difficult to evaluate the confusion, anxiety, and despair a patient might experience when his interpretation of an event is in fact accurate and the nurse contradicts him or denies the reality of the event. For this reason it is important for the nurse to be sure of her facts before she interprets a patient's statement as delusional.

A patient who was often quite delusional and hallucinating was in a cold wet sheet pack. An aide was sitting with him. In the course of their stay together the patient suddenly said, "Look at the dagger on the wall." The aide looked at the wall and saw nothing. She told the patient she didn't see the dagger. The patient became silent for five minutes and then spoke again. "Can't you hear the explosions around here?" The aide listened for a loud noise, heard nothing, and told the patient this. A short while later the patient again said, "Didn't you hear that loud explosion?" The aide listened again, heard nothing, and said to the patient, "I didn't hear anything. It must be all in your imagination." The patient became silent and noticeably more distressed until the aide left for lunch.

At lunch with other personnel, the aide heard someone comment about a distant rumbling noise that had been heard in parts of the hospital, which was due to excavating for a road under construction nearby. On pursuing the subject, the aide learned that there had, in fact, been several explosions during the time she was sitting with the patient. Recognizing her error, the aide went back to the patient after lunch. She apologized to him and told him he was right about the explosions, that there had been several of them during the time they were together, and that she simply hadn't heard them when he did.

The aide discovered, in discussing this incident with another aide, that because the patient had hallucinated a dagger on the wall she had assumed that he was also hallucinating about the explosions. This incident brought home to her in a dramatic way the importance of validating her own perceptions before denying the accuracy or validity of the patient's.

The nurse's response to the patient's autistic behavior or statements can vary greatly, depending upon how certain she is that he is distorting the environment and how accurate her knowledge is of the real situation. In some situations, the patient is quite clearly hallucinating and delusional; in others, there may be doubt; in still others, the patient may be accurate in his interpretation and the nurse wrong in her evaluation of reality. If the nurse is sure that the patient's belief is false, she can contradict it or disagree with it as, for example, when he insists that a particular nurse is trying to murder him. In other situations, she might tell the patient clearly and simply the nature of the real situation, if she knows it. For example, when the patient tells the nurse he had a visit from the Prime Minister of England yesterday, the nurse can tell him that this could not be so. Or she might try to plant a seed of doubt in the patient's mind by saying, "I know that's the experience that you feel you had, but don't you think that's quite unusual?" In some situations an appropriate way to disagree with the patient's misinterpretations might be to say, "That's the way you see it, but I see it differently," or "I know you experience it as real, but I don't hear or see the same things you do." Sometimes when the patient is hallucinating or delusional, it might be useful for the nurse to indicate that the voices he hears and the false beliefs he has are part of his mental illness; as for example, when the patient says there is a big hole in his head and the nurse can read his thoughts, or that his voices tell him to walk through the wall. In situations where the accuracy of the patient's belief or perception is in doubt, the nurse might leave the way open for their discovering together what is accurate. When the nurse and patient disagree on what they see, it might be useful for the nurse to indicate that she is trying to understand how the patient sees the situation, or why he believes as he does, even though she disagrees with him. If her relationship with the patient is good, she even might be able to discuss their differences and the reasons for these differences in the way each of them sees a situation. In disagreeing with a patient's delusion it is useless to argue with him about it or to try to convince him that he is in error. Arguing with him may only make it necessary for the patient to defend his delusion and may reinforce his conviction in his false belief. The response that is appropriate in any particular situation is difficult to know in advance; it depends on the nature of the patient's autistic behavior and on the relationship the nurse has with him. However, in rejecting a patient's misinterpretation it is important not to reject him. In the next example a nurse and the sociologist show their interest in and concern for a patient while at the same time they disagree with her delusional statements.

MRS. BARKER: The patient was talking about her brain being pulverized, that it was being sliced so the various sections could be studied. Another thing she said "they" did was to put so much pressure on her that she couldn't sleep. They had gotten her so that she had to lie in bed, cover her head, and stay away from people. Any time a nurse came near her she might be hypnotized. When I asked her why the nurses would be doing this to her, she said there was a gang of them straight from Germany. She said underneath their pleasant faces they were actually beasts and butchers.

SOCIOLOGIST: It's hard to make out what she's driving at.

MRS. BARKER: I listened to her for over an hour and I questioned her about it. She kept asking me, "Do you believe this?" I said I didn't believe it but I was interested in hearing what she had to say. She said, "Sit there and listen, then." So I sat and listened some more.

SOCIOLOGIST: Let me tell you how I handled her when she talked that way, especially about what the butchers were doing to her. I said, "I can't make out what you're talking about. Something is bothering you. There must be some connection between what you're saying and what's bothering you, but I can't figure it out. That is the way you see it about the personnel, but I'd like to tell you about the way I see it." She went on in her delusional way, and at one point she stopped and said, "OK, I'll listen to the way you see it." I tried to tell her I knew the personnel and I knew they weren't cruel. She said she thought everybody around here was inhuman, but at times I looked human. I think you can break through her delusional material for a short time, and she can listen to you. I am not sure that this is the best way, and I don't think that my talking to her made much of an impression on her delusional system at the time, but doing this frequently may have some effect.

MRS. BARKER: If patients are delusional I never argue with them, and I don't agree with them. If they ask me what I think it is, I say, "It's part of the way you feel about yourself. You must be feeling terrible." I try to maintain a good relationship with the patient be- cause I think it's exceedingly important to have a good relationship if you're going to question his delusions.

What is the effect of denying or disagreeing with a patient's delusions or distortions? Taking issue with his interpretations may have no effect, or little noticeable effect, on his false beliefs, ideas, or perceptions at a particular time or in any one situation. However, this does not necessarily mean that there may not be a cumulative effect on the patient's autistic behavior. Although the giving up of a delusional idea is not easily accomplished, some change may be effected if the nurse denies the patient's delusions in a context of personal acceptance of him, repeatedly points out reality to him without "pushing it down his throat" or arguing with him, and consistently tries to deal realistically with him. In this way the patient may be helped to modify his distortions and to maintain them with less rigidity, and his difficulty in relating to others because of these distortions may be significantly reduced.

At times, rejecting a patient's delusion may be very distressing to him. Furthermore, the nurse's way of rejecting the delusion may also add to the patient's disturbance. It is important for the nurse to recognize that although the patient's belief is false, the pain he may experience because of the belief is quite real and acute, as in the example that follows.

The nurse came into the room of a delusional patient, who was very much preoccupied with "death and killing," and stepped on a pin lying on the floor. The patient screamed, "What have you done?" The nurse was quite surprised and did not know what the trouble was. The patient said, "You've stepped on a friend of mine." The nurse felt inclined to laugh at this but did not do so. Instead, she dismissed the patient's statement lightly, as if it were of no consequence. The patient became very upset and started shaking the nurse and clinging to her. At this point the nurse realized how important this incident was. She reported later that she felt as if the patient were holding onto her to keep from drowning. The nurse said, "I then felt cruel to have dismissed her delusion about the pin so flippantly. I realized later how important it was to her."

If the nurse responds to the patient's intense feelings connected with his delusions as if these feelings are not important, or if she reacts with scorn or laughter, this will only make the patient feel unworthy and lower his self-esteem. In addition, it will emphasize the difference and distance between them. Thus, the patient may be made to feel more alone and isolated in his private world, unable to reach the nurse, and incapable of communicating with her or making himself understood.

Despite the nurse's efforts or wishes, some of her behavior might contribute to a patient's misinterpretations. One of the commonest ways in which this happens is that the patient interprets a nurse's restriction of his behavior as, "The nurse is against me." This kind of misinterpretation is inevitable in the nurse-patient relationship but gradually may be corrected as the nurse and patient develop mutually satisfying relations. In the following example the patient's behavior necessitates behavior from a nurse that "proves" to the patient that she is being persecuted by personnel.

> Miss ALLEN: Miss Jackson attacked a student at occupational therapy and was excluded from the O. T. shop. I asked the patient why she was attacking personnel. She replied, "They are trying to crush me into nothing. What's the use of having intelligence if you can't use it against them? They can object to anything I do, even to breathing. They have the keys in their power and they are trying to make nothing out of me. If I object to their objections I am in the wrong and I get blamed." I suggested that perhaps she misinterpreted what they were doing. I gave her an example of a patient shrinking as if the nurse were going to hit her when all she wanted to do was brush something off her. She thought about this but didn't reply. I then asked why she thought personnel were attacking her.

She said, "The personnel are trying to destroy me because they are jealous of me. They are jealous of my talent, my intelligence, and my health. Because of this jealousy they are trying to tear me down to their level."

A little while after this conversation Miss Jackson asked a student nurse for a cigarette. When the student held out the lighter for her, the patient attacked her. I asked Miss Jackson about it after the incident and she said, "The student was trying to put her hands in my face; she wasn't acting with respect." I saw the whole incident, and the student was obviously doing no such thing. Miss Jackson's cigarette privileges were taken away as a result of this attack, and I'm sure she interpreted this as more evidence of the fact that personnel were persecuting her.

In addition to denying them, there are other ways of handling a patient's delusions. The nurse might try to reassure the patient or indicate her sympathetic concern for him.

MRS. COOMBS: When I was with Helen today she talked a lot about people killing her or trying to kill her and said something about trying to kill other people first. She's always saying, "They don't want me; they are going to try to kill me."

SOCIOLOGIST: What do you say to her?

MRS. COOMBS: When she goes on talking that way I don't know what to say. Sometimes I put my arm around her and say, "I'm sorry, but I can't understand what you're talking about." Then sometimes she'll go on to something else that makes a little more sense. But I have found out that most of the time if the situation arises where I don't know what to say to her, the best thing to do is just to keep quiet, and she'll start talking about something else. Sometimes I question her about the names of people she's talking about. Sometimes it goes over her head or she doesn't even hear me, but other times she will answer.

SOCIOLOGIST: The more you can get some realistic answer, even a little piece of one, the better it is.

MRS. COOMBS: Today she was talking as if she had just arrived — as though she didn't know anything about the place.

SOCIOLOGIST: It might be helpful to say, "Don't you remember I talked with you yesterday and the day before?" Try to give her some idea of the continuity of your relationship.

Sometimes the patient reveals the struggle he is having with the suspicions that are part of his delusions. If the nurse is aware of the divided feelings the patient is experiencing, she may be able to understand the conflict he is in.

> MRS. BARKER: It was interesting to watch Mr. Smith the other day. He keeps saying everyone is so wicked that nobody can do anything for him. He had a cigarette in his mouth and I lit a match, and then I could see his hesitancy. First he starts to put his face forward as if to let me hold the match to the cigarette, then he pulls back again. You can see the struggle clearly—am I friend, am I foe? Am I going to burn him? Can he let me do this for him? Am I one of the torturers who's going to stick it in his face?

In many instances the nurse may have to accept the fact that she simply cannot find out the meaning of a patient's action (for example, inappropriate giggling) or the significance of a delusional belief. The patient himself may not know what is behind the giggling or his belief, or he may not be able or want to tell the nurse. In these situations, persistent questioning of the patient may make him more withdrawn or make him feel more futile and inadequate in answering the nurse. The nurse's recognition that some of these delusional ideas cannot be formulated into words by the patient and that there may be more than one meaning attached to his action may lessen her concern about discovering the real significance of the patient's misinterpretation, or what he "really means."

Some patients who show confusion along with their autistic behavior sometimes can be helped to see reality more clearly by a simple statement of the facts: for example, stating the length of time the nurse has known the patient, recalling some of the subjects they have discussed previously, pointing out some of the agreements they have arrived at in the past, or telling the patient how long it has been since their last visit. The things we take for granted about time, place, persons, and our experiences are the very things the patient distorts, misinterprets, and misunderstands. The nurse might systematically and carefully try to examine the things she, but not necessarily the patient, takes for granted. After this kind of examination she can then try to discover the best ways of communicating to the patient how she and others look at these evaluations, interpretations, and occurrences that are taken for granted.

Whenever the nurse tries to put her relation with the patient into the kind of time scale we use, and whenever she defines the patient's actions and relations with others in terms of our conventional ideas of time, she might be helping the autistic patient. For example, greeting the patient with "good morning," and, when leaving in the evening, with "good night," mentioning the time of day when appropriate, dating occurrences by the day of the week and the month of the year, all may help to orient the patient. Trying to tie up specific events in the patient's life on the ward with specific dates might also be helpful. A clear distinction between yesterday and today can be made by recalling to the patient what he and the nurse did together on each of these days. For some patients it might be helpful to tell them, and to repeat from time to time, that they are in a mental hospital, that you are a nurse, and that there are other patients like themselves on the ward. The nurse might tell a patient, "We're going to change your bed, give you a bath, and dress you," before she actually does these things, in order to emphasize the reality of these concrete happenings as well as to show her respect for the patient by informing him of what she is planning to do with and for him. When leaving a patient, telling him when you will return and returning at that time or explaining any delay may help orient him to "our reality." If these statements and actions on the part of the nurse are made in an appropriate way they may provide the experiences and the bases for an alteration in the patient's autistic behavior.

THE PATIENT'S PREOCCUPATION WITH HIMSELF

The patient may manifest his autistic behavior by deep concentration or preoccupation with himself. At these times he may be occupied with many fantastic thoughts, or he may believe that world-shattering events are about to occur which can be forestalled if he concentrates very hard or tries to hold them back with his thoughts. When the patient is in such periods of deep preoccupation, the nurse may come to believe that she can't reach him. Such a conviction may prevent her from figuring out ways of making contact with him or may prevent her from trying to do so. Even if repeated attempts have failed to break through

the patient's wall of self-concentration, it is important for the
nurse to continue to try to bring him back to reality. When a
patient is preoccupied, the nurse's problem is to get his attention
and then to hold it. Often, through activity on an elementary
level the nurse is able to reach a patient who is deeply preoccupied with himself.

MISS DENNISON: When I went in to see her, she just stared at me.
I couldn't even get her attention. I wasn't even sure she knew who I
was. She was in bad shape. I spent most of the day with her. I bathed
her and dressed her, but I couldn't break through her preoccupation.
She didn't eat anything except the food I put in her mouth. In order
to get her to do anything I had to take hold of her and practically
push her. I had to take her to the bathroom, because she couldn't
hear a word I said. I would take hold of her and make my presence
known, and then she'd say, "What?" Then I could talk to her for
a minute. I had to say about seven times, "Please listen to me for a
minute." Finally, she looked at me and said, "My God, do you know
how sick I am?" And I said, "Yes, I do. I'll stay with you. I won't go
away. Somebody will be with you, you don't have to worry about
that." Then she looked at me and I really got her attention and she
said, "I'm so upset. You don't know what it is to go through all this."
Then she talked about her life and about people who were frauds.
She looked right at me and said, "My God, am I a fraud?" She
talked a lot about herself, that she was such a little girl and she was
so scared, and this was the first time she had really come out and said
something about herself that wasn't psychotic. After I talked to her
she settled down and got into bed and was quiet.

We have found that using a physical gesture, such as taking the
patient's hand, shifting your body in relation to him, emphasizing
your presence through sound or movement, or catching his eye, is
sometimes effective with a preoccupied patient. For example, in
the illustration that follows a patient, sitting with a group of
patients who were singing, periodically got a faraway look in her
eyes, indicating that she was concentrating on her inner world.
An aide tells how he brought the patient back to participation
with the group.

MR. GATES: She would be singing and then all of a sudden she
would stop singing and stare off into space. When she went away
from the group like this, I didn't say, "Joan, sing," or "Listen to the
music," but I looked at her or tried to catch her eye.

SOCIOLOGIST: What did you do when you caught her eye?

MR. GATES: I would just change positions in front of her, get in her line of vision, smile, or something. A couple of times I said, "Hi," and looked at her quite intently, and then she would be right back singing.

We sometimes learn much about dealing with these situations in which the patient shows autistic behavior from patients who have improved and are afterward able to tell the personnel what was helpful to them. In the account that follows the patient had been delusional and hallucinating during one period of her illness. At the time she related this to the nurse, she had improved considerably and was able to talk about her behavior and the nurses' actions with her. A nurse reports the conversation.

MISS ALLEN: Miss Line was in pack and in seclusion much of the time during the two months she was on the ward. She said she has very little memory for many of the things that happened. She picked out the things she remembered, and she said that one thing she thought we all should know, that nurses ought to know, is that when a patient is terribly sick she misidentifies. She said that someone would come in whose face would remind her of somebody else, and she would take an immediate liking or disliking to this person. She said that when she would show this, personnel would seem to take it personally, and she felt that they held it personally against her, and then she would feel guilty. There were some people that didn't do this, and then after they stayed with her a long time, it would clear up in her own mind that they weren't really those people. And she said that some attendants around here say, "We don't take that stuff [hostility] from you," and she said that if it was somebody she didn't like, she was very frightened and thought, "What are *they* doing here?" She said that the patient feels it, and I think they do!

SOCIOLOGIST: The patient feels what?

MISS ALLEN: "What are they doing here? How did they know I was here?"

SOCIOLOGIST: The personnel could say, "I'm not the person you think I am."

MISS ALLEN: The thought that would go through her mind was, "How did they know I was here? What are they doing here now? They're here to torment me." Then she would scream at them— "Get out of here, you filthy thing!"—to which they would immediately react personally. I feel that if you're going to be a psychiatric nurse, you *have* to tolerate a lot of this stuff at first. The minute a patient says, "You filthy old thing," you don't say, "I don't like that," because you have no idea why the patient is saying this. And Miss Line said that long afterward she still held the same sort of feelings toward these people that she had at first. She misidentified them, and it took her a long time to figure out why and how she originally got to disliking them and they her.

SOCIOLOGIST: How would she suggest that you handle the situation? Did you ask her?

MISS ALLEN: Yes. I asked her if she ever told the personnel that they reminded her of somebody, and she said yes, that she did, and they would explain that they weren't the person, but telling her didn't do any good at that particular point. But she said that the ones that she overcame this with were those who came back again and again and again. She explained that she did want them to be kind, but firm. I told her I wanted her to know just how much I appreciated her telling me this, because it wasn't exactly a pleasant thing to discuss. Another thing that she thought we ought to know is that when personnel would come in and say, "What are you doing that for?" it would always make her worse, because she'd think, "Well, gee, I really must be sick." She said she would tear her clothes off and they'd say, "What in the world did you do that for?" She said that she would have a very good reason for what she did. She said that there were any number of reasons: that she took off her clothes because she was full of electricity and she felt that her clothes were nylon and wool and that she might catch on fire. She just *had* to get them off, and then they'd ask, "Well, what in the world are you doing that for?" Nothing made sense then. She said, "You know, to get on the disturbed ward you have to have lost faith in yourself and everybody else or you wouldn't be there! Then they come in and question your behavior, and it makes you feel even crazier." She said that some of them would say, "That's not necessary. That's just a lot of crazy stuff!" This would really take all the wind out of her sails, and then she would feel that there wasn't any point to it all.

SOCIOLOGIST: What would she rather have heard in that situation?

MISS ALLEN: I asked her about that, but she couldn't tell me. She just felt that they were questioning or reprimanding or restricting her. There wasn't anybody who understood, and she said that the things that did help were the things that were useful, like giving her milk and saying, "You need something more to drink," and like coming in and seeing her and *being* there.

SOCIOLOGIST: Now, if she throws her clothes off, you might say, "You must be terribly frightened."

MISS ALLEN: Or I was thinking that maybe you could ask, "Is there anything I could get you that you *could* wear?" It was apparent to me that by tearing off her clothes she was saying, "These clothes won't do." We could ask her if there is anything that she wanted to wear. At one point she said, "If I only had some cotton pajamas," instead of the nylon pajamas.

She asked me if I thought it was good to hire people with foreign accents—which is another interesting thing. She said that two people up there had foreign accents, and that for a long time she thought she must be in a foreign country. She said that these people talked with such an accent that she didn't really know where she was. This is the sort of confusion that we can hardly imagine.

She also said she'd like to have the person whom she responds to well, be with her. She said that the minute someone got along well with her she was taken away. She thought that maybe the reason was so that she could learn to get along with everyone. But that was pretty hard on her. She felt that you shouldn't have too many contacts with too many different people, that you should have a few who make continued contact with you so that you could get used to them and expect them to be with you. But she doesn't think a patient should rely on just one person. She had the constant fear that if that particular person left, there wouldn't be anyone; for that reason she thought it was better to have several rather than just one.

She had the idea that the food was bitter and she felt it was poisoned. She thought that it would be very helpful if four patients could eat together, then she would see other patients eating what she was asked to eat. She said, "I don't think it would have hurt the nurses to sit down and eat with me. Then you'd be sure." And another thing, she was *sure* that everything was poisoned because she was in the seclusion room next to the bathroom and she heard a lot of patients vomiting in there and having diarrhea, and it confirmed her fears. When she asked what was wrong with those patients, she would be told that they had the flu or something.

Then she told me about the beds. She said that this was one of the things that they told her was crazy on her part. She would get in bed and push it around the room with her hands, push it out from the wall and scoot it about, and the reason she did this was that a friend of hers had fallen downstairs, just as she had, had broken her back, and was an invalid for the rest of her life. And she [the patient] had hurt her back badly and it still hurt, but she didn't tell anybody about it. She was afraid that she might become bedfast. But if she could move the bed into about three different positions in the room she felt that at least she wouldn't be in exactly the same place all her life.

SOCIOLOGIST: Nobody asked her why she did this?

MISS ALLEN: No, nobody asked her why she did it. Everyone just told her that she had to leave the bed where it was.

SOCIOLOGIST: She thought she might have explained why if anyone had asked?

MISS ALLEN: I asked her that. She said that she couldn't say. She sort of thought she was so worried about her back, and yet nobody was concerned about it, that she might have told the nurses if they had asked her. She was afraid that her back was broken and that she might become bedfast.

These situations in which the patient shows autistic behavior are not easy to handle in a way that will be therapeutically useful for the patient. In general, it is useful to develop a relationship with the patient in which he becomes more comfortable and more trusting of the nurse. As she continues her relationship with him, and if he is less anxious with her, the patient may find it less necessary to relate with the nurse in an autistic way. In addition, as the nurse becomes more familiar with the patient she may find that she is better able to understand him and exchange experiences with him. The difficulties the nurse encounters need not lead to discouragement if they are seen as a chance to discover more imaginative ways of participating with the patient for his benefit.

« 6 »

The Patient Has Eating Difficulties

WHEN a patient has difficulties concerned with eating—
especially when he eats very little or not at all on his own
initiative—the nurse is faced with a serious problem. Despite his
resistance she must find some way of meeting the patient's need for
food. She must fulfill her primary responsibility of ensuring that
the patient survives and does not become physically ill because of
an inadequate diet.

The patient's present difficulties in eating are, in part, a
product of his past experiences and, in part, are perpetuated by
the kinds of interpersonal relations he is now maintaining. It may
be that in his early feeding situation and in later eating situations,
instead of having experienced warmth, comfort, satisfaction, and
a feeling of being cared for, he has suffered much anxiety, frustration, and neglect. These past emotional experiences have led him
to anticipate anxiety and displeasure with people who offer him
food or with the food itself. As a result of the dissatisfaction,
unpleasantness, and difficulty that he associates with food, he eats
reluctantly, with indecision, or not at all.

What are some of the ways in which the patient's present
experiences and interpersonal relations might interfere with his
eating adequately? A patient may be upset and unable to eat
because the nurse gives more of her time to another patient than
to him. He may be reluctant to eat because he believes the food
is poisoned or because he thinks he is eating parts of people's
bodies. He may feel that he should not have food because he is
not worthy of it. He may refuse food because he dislikes the
person offering it. He may find it difficult to eat because the social
setting in which the food is served is unpleasant or distasteful to

139

him. Still another reason may be that he is served his tray last at every meal.

In this chapter we will examine some of the problems that develop when patients have difficulty eating. We discuss three types of patients: (1) the patient who does not eat on his own initiative, (2) the patient who is indecisive and resistant about eating, and (3) the patient who eats in an unconventional manner. We will not discuss other types, such as patients who overeat.

THE PATIENT WHO DOES NOT EAT ON HIS OWN INITIATIVE

The patient who does not eat on his own initiative is completely dependent upon the nurse and others for staying alive and maintaining his physical health. It is only through the persistent efforts of nursing and medical personnel that he does not starve to death. Thus, with this type of patient the nurse has a continuing problem of "getting him to eat," and she has a further problem of helping him to assume responsibility for keeping himself adequately fed.

In order to suggest some of the factors involved in dealing with these patients, we present an example of a patient who had eating difficulties for many years. We can present only a summary of the highlights of this problem, since it continued for a long period of time.

> Mr. Winn had gradually lost weight because of his continued refusal to eat. When he was offered food at mealtime, he would reject it in a number of ways. Usually, he would become upset and shout at the nurse to leave him alone. Sometimes he would say he was not hungry; at other times he seemed physically revolted by food. At still other times he would say, "I don't like the food here. I'll eat if you'll take me to a restaurant." If the nurse insisted upon his eating, he became more upset and more resistant, sometimes throwing the tray in anger. Often, patient and nurse would shout at each other, the nurse insisting that he had to eat and the patient insisting that he would not do so. Thus, at mealtimes the patient became upset and resentful because he felt nurses were trying to force him to do something he did not want to do; personnel became angry and annoyed because they had so much trouble "doing something that was for his own good."

Although he was frequently upset at mealtime, nursing personnel had no alternative but to make sure he was fed. Thus, when he refused to eat they packed and tube-fed him. Preparing him for tube-feeding occasioned even more disturbance than offering him food. He actively resisted being packed. At times he was bewildered about the reason for being packed; at other times he was fearful and screamed, "You're poisoning me! You're trying to kill me!" In the midst of the struggle the patient would plead with and try to convince the nurse to let him skip this one meal. Sometimes nursing personnel felt guilty and distressed about the patient's anguish. At other times they were exasperated, weary, and discouraged with him. In these latter moods they sometimes omitted a tube-feeding in order to avoid the tension and struggle.

There was no consistent policy about feeding the patient. Some nurses tried to coax him to eat his food when trays were served. He often tried to hide or dispose of the food to deceive the nurse into believing he had eaten. Frequently, when he had eaten a small amount, arguments developed between nurses; one nurse would say that he had eaten enough and did not have to be tube-fed, while the other would insist that he had not and ought to be tube-fed. Other nurses did not bother to offer him a tray because they expected him to refuse it. These nurses routinely tube-fed him.

The patient often showed confusion in connection with these contradictory ways of dealing with his eating problem. He could not understand why one nurse required that he eat more than a few bites in order not to be tube-fed while another accepting his eating the same amount of food without insisting on a tube-feeding.

Because of his gradual loss of weight, nursing personnel became increasingly concerned about him. His problems in eating were discussed frequently, and at one conference a definite plan was formulated for handling the patient. It was decided that he should be tube-fed regularly until he reached his normal weight, and no attempt should be made to persuade him to eat food from his tray. It was hoped that this approach would eliminate some of the struggle, as well as the conflicting approaches of different nurses. When the patient was told about the plan, he protested that no one asked him for his opinion. Nurses agreed that this was true but told him that he had no choice about eating; they told him they were concerned about his weight and that he would be fed regularly to prevent him from becoming ill. They also said that he would be included in future planning for his own care and given a choice about the kind of responsibility he would like to take in feeding himself. At the time that the plan was initiated, nurses also changed their approach to the patient. Instead of fighting or arguing with him when he protested the tube-feeding, they tried to handle him in a matter-of-fact way. When he desperately asked, "Why are you doing this to me?" they replied, "Because we want to take care of you."

A few weeks after the initiation of the plan there was a marked decrease in the patient's anxiety and disturbance around eating. The struggles between the patient and personnel were fewer and less severe. There were, of course, ups and downs, with the patient putting up stronger protests at one time than at another, but on the whole the patient was less resistant to being fed and gained considerable weight. When he reached his normal weight, a second phase of the plan was initiated: The patient was to be offered food, and the amount he ate was to be recorded. If it was sufficient, he was not to be tube-fed. The plan was discussed with the patient; he was given some choice about where, with whom, and what kind of food he wanted to eat. In this phase of the plan, the patient again had difficulty. He constantly asked whether he would be tube-fed if he did not eat. The nurses replied firmly that he would be, and he was consistently tube-fed when his food intake was insufficient. Personnel tried to make the circumstances at mealtime as pleasant as possible for him. For a few weeks the patient ate hesitatingly and without relish, but most of the time managed to eat enough and was not tube-fed. Personnel took more interest in the patient; some nurses became quite friendly with him and stayed with him at other than mealtimes.

There were further ups and downs in the patient's eating activities. At times he did well and at other times he slipped back into previous behavior patterns. On the whole, however, he improved gradually so that at the end of a few months he was able to go to the dining room for his meals.

What were some of the factors in the situation outlined above that seemed to perpetuate the patient's difficulties about food? What contributed to the patient's gradually assuming more responsibility for feeding himself?

The frequent struggles between patient and personnel over food and tube-feeding seemed to perpetuate the patient's difficulties about eating. The idea of food, the actual intake of food, the circumstances surrounding food, and the people offering it were upsetting and anxiety-provoking for him. Thus, he resisted food, fought the personnel, and tried to defeat them, even though it meant defeating himself. Some nurses found it difficult to understand why the patient would not eat and why he fought them when they tried to feed him. Many interpreted his resistance as his *unwillingness* to eat, rather than as his *inability* to do so. Most nurses resented the burden of struggling with the patient at almost every meal, and they saw him as a constant source of trouble. The patient experienced the nurses as trying to poison him or as "doing something against him." From his point of view his resistance to tube-feeding was necessary to save his life. The nurses, on the other hand, experienced the patient as constantly in opposition to their attempts to keep him alive. It seemed that the patient's primary focus was on resisting nurses' attempts to feed him and the nurses' primary focus was on overcoming his resistance. The more each tried to accomplish his own end, the more the pattern of opposition was reinforced. Thus, at this stage the nurses' problem was to become aware of the way in which this pattern of opposition reinforced the patient's eating difficulties and to develop the kind of relationship with him that would make it unnecessary for him to oppose them by refusing to eat. In addition, in order to break the impasse, the nurses had to develop a new orientation to the situation. They had to focus on the ways in which they could help the patient eventually assume responsibility for eating adequately.

The inconsistent handling of the patient also seemed to continue his eating difficulties. Because of the hesitation, variation, and contradiction in the ways he was dealt with, he was often confused and could not understand why certain actions were taken. Because personnel were uncertain about the best way of handling him, their approach to him fluctuated. The lack of consistency and the uncertainty seemed to contribute to the patient's doubt that personnel really were concerned about him.

The patient's eating difficulties began to decrease when the nurses changed their approach, and because of this change the patient gradually became convinced that *personnel really cared about him* and that *they wanted to take care of him*. They changed their approach in a number of ways. They stopped arguing with him and arranged to tube-feed him in a consistent and efficient way. They showed an interest in him at times other than mealtime. In this way the patien did not feel that nurses were concerned about him only because they had to feed him. In addition, much of the inconsistency was eliminated by a plan for the patient that coordinated their actions. By assuming, at first, total responsibility for getting the patient fed in a systematic way, they left no doubt in his mind that *he had to eat*. By their coordination they made sure that *he ate regularly*. The elimination of personnel's indecision about how to deal with this problem seemed to relieve him.

However, in carrying out their plan personnel gave the patient the opportunity to share the initiative and responsibility in keeping himself fed. They were not content to feed him automatically and routinely but waited for the appropriate time to offer him, and to help him take some responsibility for his eating. This was accomplished by making it clear that he had no choice about whether or not he ate, but he could have a choice about where, when, what, and how he ate. Although the patient was able to take some responsibility after the plan had been in effect many weeks, he needed constant reassurance that he would be tube-fed if he did not eat. He needed the personnel to demonstrate repeatedly that *he could count on them to stop him from hurting himself*.

Just as opposition between the patient and personnel reinforced his eating difficulties, improved relations between the patient and the nurses decreased his eating difficulties. Personnel felt better about him and became more effective in dealing with him. They were able to persist in their relations with him, show a continuing interest, and maintain a consistent policy. As the patient's and staff's relations improved, the patient's eating improved; as his eating improved, their relations further improved. Thus, the patient was finally able to assume full responsibility for feeding himself.

THE PATIENT WHO IS INDECISIVE AND RESISTANT ABOUT EATING

Some patients may not refuse to eat but show such indecision and resistance about eating that they do not get an adequate amount of food. These patients present difficulties for the nurse because in order to ensure that they get enough to eat she has to discover how to deal appropriately with their indecision and resistance. An indecisive patient is presented in the following example. Mr. Jackson showed indecision about many matters, especially about eating. When offered food he could not decide whether to eat at all, how much he should eat, and what he should and should not eat. A nurse described the patient:

MISS BERRY: It's getting so I can't go near him at mealtime. I'll serve him a tray and he immediately says: "What shall I eat first?" His voice gets louder until he's practically screaming: "Should I eat this or shouldn't I? Please tell me what to do! Shall I swallow this? Will I be hurting somebody if I do? Please tell me what to do! I can't eat unless you tell me what to do!"

At mealtime the patient became upset when he was asked if he would eat or told he would have to make his own decision about eating. He pleaded with the nurses to tell him what to do, but they refused to do so. One nurse explained the reason for her refusal.

MISS BERRY: I don't think he should have to be told what to do. If we do that, he'll never be able to do anything for himself. He knows how to eat. He'd just become more and more dependent until we'd be doing everything for him the rest of his life.

Because of his fear and hesitation about eating, Mr. Jackson gradually ate less and less. As personnel insisted he make his own decisions, he became more indecisive; the more they insisted he make up his own mind, the more frantic and desperate he became in his demands to be told what to do. Sometimes personnel managed to get him to eat something, but it was so little that he continued to lose weight. He was at the point of being tube-fed when one nurse suggested a plan that she thought might help him. She expressed herself to her colleagues as follows:

MISS SMITH: Why don't we try telling him to take a bite of meat and then a bite of potato and see what happens. What we have been doing hasn't helped him. If he still can't manage to eat after we've given him directions, we might just put the spoon in his mouth and offer to feed him. I don't see why this would have to mean that he will never eat by himself or make decisions for himself. I think he needs to have this done for him before he will do anything for himself.

At lunchtime Miss Smith brought Mr. Jackson's tray into his room. When he asked her if he should eat the food, she told him to do so. She also told him that he would not hurt anyone if he ate. When he still hesitated, she took a spoonful of food and put it to his mouth. The patient took the spoon from her and began feeding himself, and the nurse sat with him while he ate. She reported her experience to the other personnel, and many of the other nurses decided to approach the patient in the same way. For a few weeks nursing personnel continued to tell the patient to eat, but he was not spoon-fed. His indecision diminished gradually, and at the end of two months he was eating in the dining room.

The patient later told a nurse that it was Miss Smith's telling him it was all right to eat and her willingness to spoon-feed him if necessary that had helped him to eat by himself.

In the illustration above, nursing personnel were reluctant to make decisions for the patient. They were uncomfortable with him and annoyed at his insistence that they make these decisions. They justified their refusal on the grounds that they did not want to continue the patient's dependence upon them. The patient continued to insist, and personnel continued to refuse. In this way the patient's indecision and his inability to eat were reinforced. When the nurses were able to change their attitude toward the patient and their way of handling him, his indecision and eating difficulty began to diminish. In this situation, *telling the patient to eat and assuming responsibility for spoon-feeding him* was a *necessary first step before the patient could make his own decisions about eating*. The appropriateness of this action was later verified by the patient's improvement and by the patient's statement of its usefulness to him. Before he could eat by himself he had to develop some trust in the nurse; he needed to know that *the nurse wanted him to eat*, that *she really cared whether he ate*, that *she wanted him to live*, and that *she was willing to make an effort to make sure he did*.

Although the nurse had to take the initiative and responsibility before the patient could make a decision for himself, she was alert to transfer this responsibility to the patient as soon as he indicated he was ready for it; that is, she let him eat by himself when he took the spoon from her hand. Thus, patients who are indecisive about eating might need an initial sign from the nurse to convince them that it is all right for them to make their own decisions and that they are worthy enough to be fed and to continue to live.

One of the ways patients show their resistance to eating is to spend a long time over food. When the patient lingers over his food, it is easy for the nurse to become annoyed and resentful. She has to see that many patients are fed and has a limited amount of time in which to do it. A routine for eating has been established, and the patient who eats slowly interferes with this routine. He requires extra time and attention which the nurse may feel she cannot give him. Under the pressure of getting her work done in the allotted time the nurse finds it difficult to remember that the patient *has to eat as slowly as he does*. If she pushes him to eat faster, he might become more resistant and eat even more slowly. If she takes his food away from him before he is finished, he might struggle with the nurse; or he might become indifferent and develop more difficulty in eating. If the nurse concentrates only on accomplishing her routine and disregards the patient's need to eat at a slow pace, she might find that eventually she is forced to spend more time with him. For if he is not permitted to eat at his own pace, he may not eat at all and require tube-feeding. Thus, if the nurse could give the slow patient the time and attention he needs, she might thereby form the kind of relationship with him that would make it possible for him to change the way he eats.

Patients also show their resistance to eating in other ways. At times a patient might cause a disturbance, upset other patients, and arouse the nurse's anger. The nurse then becomes preoccupied with handling the disturbance, and the patient is able to avoid eating. Sometimes a patient will hide food, give it away, try to persuade the nurse to let him skip a meal, or bargain with her about the amount of food he has to eat. The nurse may react to this by trying to coax or bribe him to eat. Though a patient's resistance to eating may take different forms, he is attempting by this behavior to communicate that some of his other needs are not being met. If nursing personnel could discover and meet some of his other needs, he might be less resistant at mealtime.

The Patient Who Eats in an Unconventional Manner

There are a number of ways in which patients who eat unconventionally make other patients and personnel uncomfortable. For example, a patient may mix up his food on his plate and play with it, grab food from other people's plates, and handle other people's food or drop it on the floor. In the illustration that follows a nurse describes her reaction to a patient's unconventional eating.

> Miss James: I just can't stand it when Miss Draper spits out her partially chewed food. She makes me sick when she drools, hangs onto the food, stuffs it into her mouth, or gulps it down greedily. If she were two years old I could understand it, but she's a grown woman and doesn't have to eat that way.

It is important for nursing personnel to recognize their reactions to these unconventional ways of eating. They might discover that by becoming disgusted with the way the patient eats and rejecting or punishing him because of it they may reinforce his difficulties and bring about even more serious problems about eating.

Since eating is a basic biological necessity, the relations the patient has with others in the eating situation are extremely important. Helping the patient with his eating is one way the nurse has of sharing an activity with him that is meaningful to him and vital to his welfare. Feeding a patient or helping him eat may be a way of relating to him that will not only help in the eating situation but may lay the foundation for his future satisfying relations with others. In the feeding-eating situation the nurse can take care of the patient and show that she really cares about him. In the same way that the relationship of the patient with the person offering him the food is important in increasing or decreasing his eating difficulties, the manner in which the meal is served and the circumstances under which it is served also are important. If a patient has difficulty in eating, unappetizing food served in an unattractive way under tense conditions might only serve to reinforce his difficulty. Thus, the nurse's job is to discover and try to eliminate the conditions and circumstances that reinforce the patient's difficulties about eating. Part of her role is to help the patient find ways of deriving satisfaction in the eating situation and help him assume full responsibility for maintaining an adequate diet.

The Patient Is Incontinent

OCCASIONALLY some patients on a mental hospital ward become incontinent and remain so for a long period of time. They soil their clothes, their bed, the floor, or themselves instead of using the bathroom for elimination. Some of these patients are incontinent because a physiological defect makes it impossible for them to control their bladder or bowels. Some are incontinent because of emotional problems. We shall be concerned in this chapter only with patients who are incontinent for reasons other than physiological disability.

Why does a patient become incontinent in a particular situation, and why does he continue to be incontinent? In some situations the reason seems obvious; in other situations the reason may be difficult to determine. A patient's incontinence may be related to his past history, to the anxiety he experiences concerning elimination of waste materials, to emotional needs, to his present feelings and attitudes about himself and others, to his present relations with others and to their attitudes toward him, and to other aspects of the social situation on the ward. At certain times and in certain situations, it becomes necessary for him to engage in this infant-like behavior. Exactly how this emotional process works "inside the patient" is difficult to specify. It is also difficult to understand why the patient selects incontinence as a means of expressing himself, rather than assaultiveness, demandingness, withdrawal, sexual activity, or any other pattern of behavior. But we do know that the patient's emotional life and behavior are influenced by those around him and that incontinence may be precipitated by the attitudes and reactions of personnel to the patient. Therefore, we shall focus here on those personnel reactions and social situations that contribute to patient incontinence.

One of the authors made an intensive study[1] of the circumstances under which patients became incontinent. He found that patients who are regularly incontinent over a considerable period of time are incontinent, in part, because of the way nurses relate with them. This does not mean that the nurse is to be blamed for the patient's incontinence. It means, rather, that some of the attitudes, feelings, and activities of nursing personnel encourage, provoke, or reinforce those feelings in the patient that lead to his incontinence. If the nurse can become aware of her effect on the patient, she may be able to change her way of relating with him and thus make it unnecessary for him to continue his incontinent behavior.

What are the patient's feelings before and while he is incontinent? What is he trying to tell us with this behavior? When he is incontinent, the patient is often *anxious and insecure;* he may feel helpless and want someone to take care of him. One way to achieve this is to engage in infant-like behavior. This does not necessarily mean that the patient deliberately becomes incontinent. The whole process may go on automatically, outside the patient's awareness.

At the time the patient becomes incontinent he may feel he is *not worthwhile.* When the patient thinks little of himself and feels disgusted with himself he seeks a means of expressing his feeling of low self-esteem. One way of doing this is to be incontinent—to perform an act that will lower him in other people's eyes and show how disgusting he really is. Because he has a low opinion of himself, the patient may feel that he is incapable of behaving in other than an unpleasant and distasteful way.

A patient may feel *lonely and isolated* when he becomes incontinent. It is difficult for him to ask for companionship in a direct way; therefore, he uses an indirect way of getting the nurse's attention. When he soils himself, the nurse will come to clean him.

[1] Schwartz, Morris S., and Alfred H. Stanton, "A Social Psychological Study of Incontinence," *Psychiatry*, vol. 13, November, 1950, pp. 399–416.

Even this brief contact with the nurse is felt to be better than continuous isolation.

Other feelings the patient may have when he becomes incontinent are *hopelessness, anger, and resentment*. When he feels hopeless, the patient does not care about himself; he feels that it is too much of an effort to use the bathroom, and that it does not matter whether he soils himself. When he is angry or resentful, he may use incontinence as a way of making those around him uncomfortable, as a means of retaliation against those who have made him uncomfortable.

Although the feelings described above are usually associated with patient incontinence, the patient may not be aware of a connection between his incontinence and these feelings. Incontinence follows as a natural response when these feelings are present, ordinarily without premeditation on the patient's part. The patient may also unconsciously use incontinence to communicate to the nurse how he feels—that he feels anxious, unworthy, lonely, hopeless, or angry and resentful. If the nurse receives this communication, she can then proceed to discover the conditions and circumstances that evoke these feelings in the patient and bring about his incontinence.

What kinds of situations precipitate the patient's incontinent behavior? What attitudes and actions on the part of the nurse contribute to its continuation? It seems that our cultural emphasis on cleanliness, toilet training, and avoidance of unpleasant odors makes it difficult for the nurse to accept incontinent behavior with equanimity or in a matter-of-fact way. She may try to conceal her negative feelings, or she may react with overt expressions of distaste, disgust, or revulsion. Her overt reaction may take any of a number of forms: She wrinkles her nose or makes a wry face when she has to clean the patient up. She insists that the patient clean up "the mess" himself. She handles the soiled clothing gingerly, holding it with two fingers as far away from her as possible. In talking with the patient she reveals her distaste and revulsion. When she rejects the patient because of his incontinent behavior, she reinforces his feelings of low self-esteem. By her disgust and revulsion she "makes him" feel repulsive, and he, therefore, continues his repulsive behavior. The patient's conscious or unconscious feeling and thoughts might be, "If that is what you think I am [disgusting], that is how I will have to be [incontinent and repulsive]."

Closely related to the nurse's disgust with the patient is her moralistic attitude toward him. The nurse may feel and say openly that the patient is "bad" for engaging in incontinent behavior, thus expressing the attitudes and judgments conventionally accepted outside the hospital. She may go even further and "bawl him out," threaten to punish him if he is incontinent again, try to shame him, or actually punish him. Such a moralistic attitude may make the patient resentful, and in defiance he may maintain or increase his incontinence. If the punishment is severe, the patient may stop his incontinence, but it may then be impossible for the nurse to form a therapeutic relationship with him. And he may become more withdrawn and more preoccupied with autistic thoughts and less accessible to others because of increased and reinforced hatred for them. Even if the nurse is not harsh with the patient, she still may feel that he has done something wrong, and may convey this in her manner, indicating directly or indirectly: "You should know better than to do this." "How could you do such a thing?" "You should behave differently." When the nurse approaches the patient with a moralistic attitude she contributes to his feeling of low self-esteem and inadequacy, and to his feeling that nobody understands him. The patient may experience a feeling of despair because no one understands that he cannot control his incontinent behavior as long as he is made to feel unworthy, inadequate, and hopeless.

One of the ways in which the nurse deals with situations of incontinence is to avoid the patient. She leaves the patient soiled for long periods of time, ignoring or remaining indifferent to the fact that he has been incontinent. She isolates the incontinent patient so that he will not be noticed and the ward will not appear unpleasant. She might recognize that he needs to be cleaned up but try to "pass the buck." These attitudes and actions on the part of the nurse reinforce the patient's loneliness and increase his resentment. When the nurse permits the patient to be soiled for a long period of time, he may feel that she does not care whether or not he is soiled. The patient might then think, "If no one cares, why should I? If no one makes an effort to keep me clean, why should I make an effort to keep myself clean?"

When the nurse does not fulfill the patient's needs—when she refuses to meet his requests, frustrates him, ignores him, and leaves him ungratified—the patient may respond with incontinent behavior. If he does not receive the attention and interest he needs and wants, he may feel he is not worthy of having his needs fulfilled. He also may continue his incontinence to show how dissatisfied he is with the way his needs are being handled.

If a patient has been incontinent over a long period of time, the nurse may come to feel hopeless about his changing this pattern of behavior. This feeling of hopelessness leads to the expectation that the patient's incontinence will continue. Because of this expectation the nurse does not even offer him an opportunity to use the bathroom. By showing what she expects of him in this way, she contributes to the continuation of his incontinence. It is difficult for the patient to change his pattern of behavior if people around him do not believe he can or will change it. Thus, the circular pattern will continue until the nurse changes her expectations.

The nurse's attitudes, expectations, feelings, and actions described above contribute both directly and indirectly to the precipitation and continuation of the patient's incontinence. This does not mean that each time these attitudes and actions are present the patient will respond with incontinence. But we found that when the patient was regularly incontinent the circumstances described above were ordinarily present. Thus, the nurse's task is to find ways of changing her relations with the patient in order to make it unnecessary for him to respond to her with incontinent behavior.

In order to contribute to the elimination of patient incontinence the nurse has to learn how to handle her attitudes and feelings and to carry on relations with the patient so as not further to lower his self-esteem, his feelings of worthlessness, anxiety, loneliness, and resentment. Stated in a positive way, this means that the nurse respects the patient and shows consideration for him as a person despite his incontinent behavior; that she accepts this behavior as part of his mental illness; and that she does not have to criticize him, moralize about it, or impose sanctions upon him. She tries to understand him and the reasons for his incontinence. She encourages the patient by indicating to him that she thinks he can do better in the future but she does not try to force him to change his behavior at the moment. In other words, the nurse supports the patient with the view that she can see the potentiality for change in him, while she also lets him know that he does not have to change immediately. In general, it seems that accepting the patient, showing respect and consideration for him despite his behavior, understanding him, and meeting his needs are prerequisites for the patient's giving up incontinence. The patient gives it up not in a deliberate or calculated way but as a natural consequence of the relationship he is having with the nurse.

It will be helpful to the nurse if she can distinguish between two types of acceptance of the patient. On the one hand, in some situations *the nurse will have to accept the patient's incontinence* before he will feel acceptable to her and accepted by her. In these situations the nurse has to handle her feelings of discomfort and resentment in such a way that she does not reject the patient by rejecting his behavior. This does not mean that the nurse pretends not to mind the behavior when she is made uncomfortable by it; rather, it means that she does not express her discomfort in such a way as to make the patient anxious and insecure. She might be able to handle her feelings more satisfactorily if she could look upon her acceptance of the patient's incontinence as temporary —until the patient feels that it is not a satisfying way of communicating or relating with others. On the other hand, there may be some patients with whom the nurse can be overt in her rejection of incontinent behavior, but *it is important that she accepts the patient though she rejects his behavior*. She may become angry when the patient soils her, or she may tell him that his messiness makes her uncomfortable, but she does this in a way that indicates she is concerned about him as well as herself. For example, a nurse who had a good relationship with a patient was distressed when she saw her urinating on the floor and wondered what she might do to help her give up this behavior. She said to the patient in a concerned manner, "What can we do for you so you won't have to keep peeing on the floor like this?" In maintaining the balance between accepting the patient while rejecting the incontinent behavior, the nurse shows respect for and takes into account both the patient and herself. She recognizes that the patient does not like having to be so unpleasant, and she helps to increase his self-esteem by rejecting the part of him and his behavior that he himself rejects. By doing this she also indicates that he can change.

In addition to respecting and accepting the patient, the nurse can undertake specific activities that might make it unnecessary for him to be incontinent. If she can anticipate when the patient might become incontinent, she may be able to give him the support he needs to make his incontinence unnecessary. This means that the nurse is familiar enough with the patient and observant enough of him to be able to detect the preliminary signs of incontinence. A nurse who was able to do this reports her experience.

> MISS ALLEN: If you watch what Blanche does, if you watch her very carefully, you can tell every time she is going to be incontinent. When she is left out of something or has been hurt or refused something, she gets frustrated. You can tell by the way she walks and the way she looks that she will be incontinent. She'll walk back to her room and wet her dress. But if you indicate that you notice what is happening and follow her into her room and stay with her, you can avoid the incontinence.

Out of these specific situations in which the nurse helps the patient refrain from incontinence, the patient may come to feel the acceptance and understanding that will help him continue to eliminate conventionally.

Sometimes the patient can be helped to stop his incontinence by the nurse's attitude that he *can stop*. This is different from saying that he "must" or "should" stop. In these situations the nurse gives the patient the kind of support that helps him do what he might want to do but cannot do by himself. For example, an aide entered a room where the patient was about to defecate on the floor. She said simply, "Maybe you don't have to do it there." The patient immediately stopped and went to the bathroom. Apparently in this situation the patient did not want to defecate on the floor and in order to refrain from doing so he needed only the aide's support that he did not have to do it.

Nursing personnel can become more fully aware of the attitudes and activities that tend to reinforce a patient's incontinence and those that help him discontinue this pattern of behavior. With this awareness they can work toward developing those interpersonal relations with the patient that will help to solve a difficult and disagreeable problem for personnel and that will be of therapeutic benefit to the patient.

·《 8 》·

The Patient's Behavior Has a Sexual Connotation

IN some situations on the ward the nurse interprets the patient's behavior as having a sexual connotation. These may be situations in which the patient makes seductive gestures toward the nurse, masturbates in her presence, invites her to have sexual intercourse with him, uses sexual words, tries to feel parts of the nurse's body, or exposes his sexual organs. Under these circumstances the nurse may become concerned about what the patient is trying to do to her or is trying to get her to do with him. She does not know how to act with the patient and finds him difficult to handle. In this chapter we discuss some possible meanings of such behavior, the nurse's reaction to this behavior, and some of the ways in which the nurse might handle these situations.

THE MEANING OF THE PATIENT'S BEHAVIOR

An obvious interpretation the nurse can make of behavior that has a sexual aspect is to attribute it to a sexual urge for which the patient is seeking gratification. It is undoubtedly true that in some of these situations the patient may be seeking some sort of sexual contact. But in many instances this may not be what he is seeking, nor is it necessarily his main objective or wish in a situation that has a sexual connotation. A number of other equally valid interpretations can be made of the patient's behavior. He may need someone to show him interest and concern. He may want a simple physical contact, to touch someone and be touched by him as an expression of friendliness and warmth. He may be asking for tenderness and acceptance in one of the few ways he can. He may be trying in an unskilled way to form some relationship with the nurse in order to reduce his isolation and loneliness. He may be trying to communicate something about himself to the nurse. He may be asking for reassurance that he is not repulsive and disliked. He may be acting out sexual fantasies that have little relation to personnel who are with him in the situation at the moment. He may be trying to find out how to manage his body in relation to someone else. He may be trying to get the nurse to notice and attend to him by engaging in behavior that he knows will attract her attention and may be startling or upsetting to her. The interpretations we have suggested by no means exhaust the possible meanings of the patient's behavior. It may have many other meanings as well as a combination of meanings, and neither the patient nor the nurse may be aware of the needs the patient is seeking to have fulfilled through this behavior.

The Nurse's Reactions

When the nurse interprets the patient's behavior as a sexual approach to her, she may react in a variety of ways. She may become embarrassed and want to get away from the patient. She may become uncomfortable and confused in her response to him. She may become angry with and critical of him and tell him that he "ought to be ashamed" of himself, that his behavior is "disgusting," or that he "should know better than to do that." She may want to punish him. She may become fearful of what is going to happen to her in the situation.

The nurse sometimes feels anxious and guilty about the patient's sexual gestures toward her. Her anxiety and guilt might arise because some sexual feeling is stimulated in her. She finds it difficult to recognize these feelings or admit to herself that she has them, because she is "not supposed" to have such feelings about patients. Denying the existence of these feelings makes it more difficult to handle them adequately. For if she is unclear about the reason for her guilt and anxiety she cannot come to grips with the source of her uneasiness. On the other hand, if she develops an awareness of her sexual feelings when they are present and accepts the fact that nurses do experience such feelings in some situations, she may be able to handle her feelings more adequately. *It might be helpful for the nurse to remember that recognizing these feelings does not mean she wants a sexual relation with the patient or that she will act on her feelings.* The nurse's personal values and professional as well as hospital limitations will help her not to act on these feelings. With a clearer awareness of them and the recognition that she will not act on them, she may not have to reject the patient because his sexual behavior makes her feel guilty about the feelings stirred up in her.

The nurse's reaction to the patient when his behavior has sexual connotations and the way she handles his behavior have an important influence on the patient. Her reactions may contribute to the continuation of the behavior or may help to modify it. Thus, it is important for the nurse to be aware of her reactions to the patient and to observe the effects of these reactions on him.

WAYS OF HANDLING THE PATIENT

There are times when the nurse's embarrassment and discomfort seem to contribute to the continuation of the patient's sexual behavior. This is illustrated in the example that follows:

> Mr. Johns [an aide] had difficulty with Miss Smith over a considerable period of time. In any contact he had with her she made suggestive remarks to him and invited him to have sexual intercourse. This behavior made him uncomfortable, and the more uncomfortable he became, the more insistent the patient became. At one time she tried to remove his trousers. He was extremely embarrassed by this and hurriedly left the patient. He then tried to avoid her because he was so distressed by her behavior. However, whenever she had an opportunity, the patient continued to make sexual gestures toward him.

In the situation described above the aide was unable to talk about the patient's behavior, either with other staff members or with the patient, because he was so embarrassed by it. He saw it only as a sexual attack on him. To avoid the patient was the only solution that occurred to him. Thus, he was unable to arrive at a satisfactory relationship with her. In some way, the aide's response seemed to encourage the patient to continue to approach him in this sexual way.

In another illustration two student nurses take different approaches to the same patient with different results.

INSTRUCTOR: I understand that you're instructed to leave Mr. Bryan's door open when you're in with him. Why is that?

MISS WILEY: Well, it's because of the things he does when we go in.

INSTRUCTOR: What does he do?

MISS WILEY: He asks one of us to come in and read to him, and then he closes the door. You start to read and pretty soon he's lying there masturbating with his pants unzipped. I get so embarrassed I have to leave.

INSTRUCTOR: Has anybody else had this experience?

MISS SEARS: I did. He did the same thing with me, but when he closed the door I left it closed. I got uncomfortable when he started to masturbate, so I just told him, "I want to stay and read to you, but when you do this I get embarrassed. I'd rather you zipped up your pants."

INSTRUCTOR: Then what happened?

MISS SEARS: He zipped them up and I went on reading. But then he started feeling my leg.

INSTRUCTOR: What did you do?

MISS SEARS: I didn't move away from him, but I said, "This is more of the same kind of thing that makes me uncomfortable. I want to stay, so please stop." He did.

INSTRUCTOR: I think it's important that you could stay with him and show him that you didn't have to reject him because of his behavior, but you also showed him that you wanted him to stop it because it made you so uncomfortable. He responded to your suggestion, so it would seem that he is more interested in having your company than in continuing to masturbate. Maybe he isn't able to control this behavior without some help from you.

MISS WILEY: He said something like that yesterday. I was playing cards with him in the living room and nobody else was around. After awhile he got up and said, "I can't stand this any more. You know, a lot of the things I do I can't help. I know you're a nurse and I'm a patient and I don't really want to act the way I do." I just stood there and didn't say anything. He suddenly grabbed me and got real close and tried to kiss me. I told him to stop and then I left the room. When I thought about it later, I realized I didn't catch on that he was saying that he just couldn't be alone with me because of what he felt like doing. Maybe I could have suggested we go into the hall.

INSTRUCTOR: That was fine that he could tell you how he felt. Maybe you can help him stop doing what he tells you he really doesn't want to do.

In the foregoing example one nurse feels threatened by the patient's behavior and has to leave and, therefore, the relationship between the nurse and patient is cut off. Another nurse is also embarrassed, but overcomes her embarrassment sufficiently to tell the patient how she feels. Her way of handling the situation may have conveyed to him that his behavior does not make him so objectionable that the nurse has to leave him; at the same time she helped him stop doing something he may not have wanted to do.

In the following illustration student nurses, graduate nurses, and an instructor talk about their different interpretations of a patient's behavior in an attempt to discover an appropriate way of handling his apparently sexual actions.

INSTRUCTOR: I hear that you have been having difficulty with Mr. Miles.

MISS AKINS: When he starts patting me and trying to kiss me, he makes me so uncomfortable that I have to get away. I wonder why he tries to embarrass us.

MISS BOYD: I don't think he tries to embarrass us. Maybe we just think his behavior is sexual when it isn't. When he tries to kiss me or rubs against me, he reminds me so much of my little cousin. He's about twelve and he comes up to his mother and does the same sort of thing. All he wants is a little affection.

MISS CLAY: You know Mr. Miles likes to have his back rubbed, but you have to set limits for him. It works if you tell him to take off his shirt, lie on his stomach, and that you'll use the lotion to rub his back. He gets quiet and relaxed after that. If you don't tell him this, he tries to get you to rub his stomach. I tried just telling him I was going to get the lotion for his back, but then he asked me to rub his stomach. I have to tell him exactly what I want him to do and what I'm going to do every time.

INSTRUCTOR: It may be he just wants to get close to you and have some physical contact. You have to set the limits each time, but he responds to this and accepts it as part of your nursing him.

MISS CLAY: He gets less tense when I rub his back, and he knows that's all I'm going to do. But some people have criticized me for doing it. They say I'm inviting sex from him. So now I tell them just what I'm going to do. I wish we could figure out what else we could do for him so people wouldn't be saying "No" to him all the time.

INSTRUCTOR: Why do you think so many people have to say "No" to him?

MISS AKINS: I do because I get so embarrassed. He tries to kiss me in front of everybody—other patients and other personnel. Sometimes he makes me really angry because he keeps on. He seems to know he can get under my skin this way. Sometimes I think he just does it to make me mad!

INSTRUCTOR: You think he behaves this way deliberately? He does it on purpose?

MISS AKINS: Yes.

MISS CLAY: I don't think he does. If you'll just do something for him, he'll respond. When he does that, I think he wants you to recognize him and be friendly to him. I think he likes to have some physical contact, but I pat him or just touch him in a warm way and that seems to be enough. I think it's important for us to show him that we understand his need for warmth and that we can respond to it. I don't think it's sex he wants at all because he stops making passes when I pat him or show him I like him. Sometimes I put my arm around his shoulder, and he doesn't do anything sexual at all after that.

INSTRUCTOR: Maybe you could approach him first instead of waiting for him to approach you. Maybe you could just reach out as you pass him and pat him on the elbow or put your arm on his and walk with him a little. He seems to be letting you know that physical contact is important and that he can accept your setting the limits.

MISS JONES: You mean if we gave something of ourselves first and let him know we understood his need for physical touching, it wouldn't have to be any more than that?

INSTRUCTOR: That might be an alternative to saying "No" all the time.

In the foregoing illustration one nurse seemed to respond exclusively to the sexual aspect of the patient's behavior. Another nurse saw it as the patient's attempt to relate with her and to get some warm response from her. Using the latter interpretation of the patient's behavior, the nurse is able to relate to him and set limits for him so that he stops his annoying and embarrassing actions. In addition, the example shows the importance of the attitudes of the nurse's colleagues. If other staff members are critical of the nurse's activities with the patient and she is anxious and uncertain about her attempts to deal with his sexual behavior in a nonsexual way, she might find it difficult to continue her relationship with him. Thus, it is important for the nurse to explain to her colleagues what she is going to do with the patient and receive some acceptance and understanding from them.

At times, the very behavior that drives a nurse away from the patient may indicate that there is promise for a good relationship between them. Because the nurse is concentrating on the sexual connotation of the behavior, she might not see that it also shows that the patient can form a constructive relationship with a nurse. This is illustrated in the following example.

A nurse was sitting on a bed with a patient, helping her sort her clothing. The patient moved closer to the nurse, started to rub her legs, and tried to feel her breasts. The nurse became embarrassed, pushed the patient away, and left the room. The patient laughed in a "silly" way when the nurse pushed her away, but did not pursue her. The nurse told other ward personnel about the incident, and some personnel described it as homosexual behavior. The nurse liked the patient and wanted to visit with her, but the patient's actions and the staff's attitude made her feel uncomfortable about doing so. Nevertheless, she went back to visit the patient. Again the patient attempted to feel parts of her body, and again the nurse became uncomfortable and quickly left the room. She expressed her discomfort and inability to handle the situation to the ward personnel. One of them suggested that the problem be discussed at a ward conference.

At the conference some thought that the behavior was homosexual and that the nurse should keep away from the patient. Others thought that the patient was trying to show her friendly feelings to the nurse, and, not knowing how to do this very well, was doing it in an awkward way. The nurse was advised to tell the patient that she felt friendly toward her and she thought the patient felt friendly, too, and that they could be friends without this "feeling" behavior. The nurse decided to follow this course. During a visit, when the patient started feeling her, the nurse said simply, "I would like to be friends with you, and this behavior isn't necessary for us to be friends." The patient stopped immediately, and after that she and the nurse formed a good relationship. Their relationship went so well that the nurse was able to take the patient shopping—something the patient was rarely able to do with anyone else.

If the nurse had been frightened away by the patient's behavior or by some of the personnel's interpretation of the patient's intentions, she would have missed the opportunity to form a worthwhile relationship with the patient, as well as to help her discontinue the sexual behavior. Her own embarrassment and some staff members' feelings that she should avoid this behavior by avoiding the patient easily could have led the nurse to reject the patient. However, by focusing on another interpretation of the patient's behavior, she was able to change her response to the patient and thus change the patient's response to her. It was important that the nurse received support from some of her colleagues, which helped her feel less guilty while she was trying to work out her relationship with the patient.

The final example illustrates how a patient's apparently sexual behavior can continue for a long period of time and become a persistent ward problem.

> Miss Berry sometimes walked around the ward nude, frequently danced and moved in a suggestive way, and "threw" herself at certain male staff members. She "wrapped herself" around these men, clung to them, kissed them, danced seductively in front of them, and asked them sexually provocative questions. Usually, they rejected her, sometimes mildly, sometimes severely. Despite these continued rejections, she persisted in her behavior. The men who were thus "attacked" and other staff members who saw her behavior were angry and resentful. Some had moralistic attitudes and called her behavior "disgusting."
>
> In trying to cope with this patient's behavior, the nurses tried warning her, bawling her out, talking with her in a rational way about it, and, finally, secluding her. They were dissatisfied with their results and discussed Miss Berry at a conference. One nurse's statement is given below.
>
> MISS ALBIE: We decided we weren't going to let her out on the ward unless she was properly clad. She would come out in her housecoat with nothing under it, and somehow the housecoat would fall open. Or she would come out in a raincoat with nothing under it, or in a blouse and skirt with the skirt always unzipped and the blouse always unbuttoned. We decided to try to make her either remain in her room or remain dressed. But somehow I never felt right about this, and I had difficulty following through with this decision. My heart really wasn't in it.

The men Miss Berry "made love to" treated her in different ways: they pushed her away or told her to "stop it." They struggled with her, became angry with her, treated her contemptuously, or tried to avoid her. None of their actions had much effect in altering the patient's behavior. The nursing staff were in great conflict about this patient and they were at a loss to know what to do with her. Seclusion was frequently tried. They agreed that limits should be set on the patient's behavior, but the kind of limits and how they should be set could not be worked out satisfactorily. At one conference the personnel were concerned with the meaning of the patient's behavior and how she felt about it. One of the doctors offered this explanation:

DR. HUGHES: She doesn't get anything out of this behavior. This is something she feels guilty about and regrets after she does it. After we've taken her away from John [one of the male aides] I've heard her call herself a "filthy whore." When she was in seclusion, she'd strip herself and masturbate. After she wrapped herself around John she went on the porch and laughed in a crazy way. Then she ran back to her room and continued the crazy laughter. These are all signs of increased anxiety. Even though it seems as if this is something she wants to do, I don't think permitting her to do it does her any good. I think we should try to limit her so she doesn't act in a way that is disrespectful to herself.

At this conference it was suggested that instead of pushing the patient away when she made advances, the male aide might put his arm around her shoulder or pat her head in a friendly fashion. It was suggested that the patient might not be interested in sex at all but merely wanted some affection. Only one male aide was able to do this. On one occasion when the patient sprawled all over him, he patted her on the head and gave her a hug in a fatherly way, very much as one would a small child who was seeking some affection. Her provocative behavior stopped with him in that situation. He repeated the friendly, warm gestures with her a few times, and in a short while her provocative behavior disappeared with him. The other men continued to be embarrassed by her and to reject and avoid her. Her sexual behavior continued with them.

The foregoing example illustrates the way in which nursing personnel can continue or reinforce patient behavior. By reacting to the behavior as if sexual activity were the only response the patient wanted, the personnel were uncomfortable, embarrassed, and guilty. As a result, they tended to isolate or avoid the patient. However, they were in conflict about such isolation. By these responses to the patient they indicated they did not understand her needs and made her feel unacceptable. The interpretation of the patient's needs only as sexual, the personnel's continued discomfort, and their rejection of her seemed to encourage the patient to persist in her behavior. On the other hand, the example also illustrates how personnel can contribute to changing the patient's behavior. When one aide was able to understand her communication and to see her behavior as expressing a need for tenderness, friendliness, a need to feel worthwhile, he was able to respond to her differently. Because of his changed response, the patient was able to respond differently to him and to give up her sexual behavior. Thus, it seems that certain actions of personnel made it necessary for the patient to continue her behavior and that other actions on their part made this behavior unnecessary.

Situations in which the patient's behavior has a sexual connotation might be easier for the nurse to handle if she were clearly aware of her own feelings and her interpretations of the patient's behavior. If the nurse believes that the patient is seeking a sexual contact, she can respond to his behavior by making the limits in the situation clear to him, but in doing so she does not have to reject the patient. *She can accept his behavior as his way of expressing himself at the time and she can try to meet some of his other needs.* Frequently, the patient is not seeking sexual activity, and the nurse's interpretation of his behavior would be more accurate if she saw it as a need for warmth, tenderness, and friendliness. If she can respond appropriately to these needs she can then show the patient that she understands him, that he matters to her, and that it is possible for him to receive a simple affectionate response from another person.

« 9 »

The Patient Is Suicidal

IN our culture it is taken for granted that each person will want to live as long as possible, will make some effort to do so, and will be helped to do so by those around him. When someone acts contrary to these cultural standards by trying to take his own life, we feel threatened and insecure. When a patient on a mental hospital ward attempts suicide, anxiety is a common and widespread reaction on the part of nursing personnel. It is understandable that such an act should be particularly anxiety-provoking for the nurse, inasmuch as one of the objectives of nursing the mentally ill is to keep the patient from hurting himself—especially to prevent a serious or fatal injury. Unlike other problems on the ward, if the patient succeeds in killing himself there is no second chance.

Because the idea of suicide arouses so much anxiety, we can expect some discomfort and difficulty on the part of nursing personnel as they think about this subject. This anxiety is unavoidable if the nurse is to develop a better understanding of situations in which the patient contemplates or attempts suicide and if she is to increase her usefulness to the patient in anticipating and preventing self-injury. In discussing these situations we will suggest some ways of looking at them that might be helpful. We will not discuss all aspects of the problem of suicide but will focus on some of the activities the nurse can undertake in order to prevent patient suicide and on the nurse's reactions when a patient has made a suicidal attempt. Our goal here, as in the other chapters, is to stimulate the nurse to think about the problem and to help the nurse find her own solutions in her own situation.

It is important to state clearly what we mean by "the suicidal patient." We refer to the patient who has given some indication that suicide is a possible course of action for him in the immediate or near future. This evidence may be present in any of the following forms: in his preoccupation with and indirectly expressed thoughts about committing suicide; in overt talk about killing himself or threats to kill himself; in preparing to injure himself by hiding sharp instruments or glass; in his general orientation and manner expressing the attitude that life is not worth living; in attempting to injure himself, whether the actual intention is to bring about his death or just to hurt himself superficially. Any of these actions, or others, may be signs that lead to the patient's eventually injuring himself seriously. It is difficult to tell by these preliminary signs when or how the talk or thoughts will turn into action—a definite attempt to end his life.

What is a patient communicating to us about his feelings when he tries to take his own life or is preoccupied with suicidal thoughts? He may be telling us (without necessarily being aware of it) that he feels living is without purpose, that his relationships with others and with himself are meaningless, that he sees no solution to his problems, and that he sees no possibility of living in anything but misery. The patient is telling us that he feels discouraged, despairing, hopeless, and incapable of doing anything to change his situation. The patient may also feel resentful, hostile, and hateful toward persons in his immediate environment, as well as toward other persons who are important to him. But he is unable to express these feelings verbally and cannot act on them by trying to injure the other person physically. Instead, he turns his hatred inward—on himself. He may feel that in trying to kill himself he will punish those who have hurt him by making them feel guilty and sorry about his death. In trying to hurt himself the patient is also telling us how terribly alone he feels, how unbearable is the pain and torture he experiences, how helpless he feels, how serious and urgent is his need to be understood, and how desperate is his need for support and help—for someone to *do something for him*. If these communications are not heard, are not understood, or are not responded to, the patient may become more frantic and even more desperate. Thus, the nurse's task is to recognize and respond to the patient's plea for help.

PREVENTION

From a long-range point of view, the most effective way of preventing suicide is to create the conditions and establish the kinds of relations with the patient that make it unnecessary for him to seek this type of solution to his problems. This means that the nurse carries on relations with the patient that contribute to his satisfaction, security, and well-being so that he does not feel completely abandoned and hopeless. If there is just one person— a nurse, for example—*who has consistently cared about the patient in the past and cares for him now*, this may be sufficient to prevent him from getting to the point where he seriously considers or actually chooses suicide as an alternative to his way of living. Their past experiences together and the patient's present feelings about the nurse might provide the background and context that eliminate this drastic action as a present possibility for the patient.

Recognizing Patient Intentions

When a patient has come to the point where suicide is a possible course of action (or, in language more commonly used, where he is a suicidal risk, a potential suicide, or actively suicidal), the nurse faces the problem of anticipating and preventing this action. In order to do this she must recognize as early as possible the signs and cues he gives that these are his tendencies or intentions.

Nurses use many cues as warnings that alert them to a patient who is becoming or has become so distressed that he contemplates suicide as a way out. These cues consist of observations of their own feelings as well as observations of the patient's actions and expressions of his feelings and attitudes. One of these cues may be the nurse's feeling of discomfort—the vague apprehension that something is wrong with the patient; or she may find that she is feeling sad or morbid without knowing why. If the nurse pays attention to this cue, focuses on it, and follows it until it crystallizes into a definite idea of what is wrong, she may discover that her uneasiness or restlessness is related to her dawning awareness that the patient is revealing to her his preoccupation with suicide or that her sadness is related to her identification with the patient. If the nurse observes the patient's activities closely enough, she may discover different patterns of behavior for different patients that indicate that they are contemplating suicide. One patient may become more and more depressed, increasingly showing that he does not feel life is worth living. Another patient may change suddenly from depression to overactivity and cheerfulness, but the nurse senses that there is something "wrong" with this sudden change. Sometimes a patient who has been overtly hostile and assaultive becomes seclusive, withdrawn, and unwilling to eat. Some patients tell the nurse indirectly and subtly that they are thinking about suicide. Other patients are direct and obvious about their intentions, talking openly about suicide, and getting and using instruments with which they can hurt themselves. How easily and quickly a nurse can become alerted to the cues is in large part dependent upon her familiarity with the patient and the care with which she makes her observations. If she knows the patient and is an alert observer, she may be able to notice early significant changes in patient behavior and to receive the patient's communication about his suicidal intentions.

In the example below the nurse did not recognize two slight changes in the patient's behavior which she might have taken as cues that he was thinking about committing suicide that night.

> A depressed patient had been preoccupied with himself and had not participated in ward activity for two or three weeks. When offered reading material he would refuse it. One day he asked the nurse to get him a certain book of poetry from the library. Upon receiving the book that evening he became absorbed in it and continued to read it avidly all evening. The poems dealt with death, destruction, and other morbid subjects. At bedtime the nurse offered him the sedation that he had been taking regularly, and he refused it. The nurse did not question his refusal nor did she suspect that anything was wrong because of it. In the early hours of the morning the patient attempted suicide.

In thinking about the situation described above, the nurse felt that his preoccupation with the morbid poems and his refusal of sedation should have been a signal to her to observe the patient more carefully, to spend more time with him, and to increase her precautions with him.

In the following example the patient indicates her suicidal preoccupations to the nurse, and the nurse "catches on."

> MISS ALLEN: Claire wrote a letter to her father today which she gave me and didn't seal, and I read it. In it she said that leaving her in this hospital meant a slow and terrible death—in fact, that she was already dead and was just waiting to get out of here to make this an accomplished fact. I think this could be interpreted as a suicidal threat. I would suggest that we keep an eye on her. She can send sealed letters to her father, so when she sends an unsealed one it's as though she is saying, "Take a look at what's in here."

In the situation presented above the nurse readily recognizes the initial cue—the unsealed letter—as a sign that the patient wants to tell her something. When she follows through on this cue she discovers the patient's thoughts about suicide.

Sometimes the nurse does not recognize the signs the patient gives or hear what he is trying to tell her. At these times the patient may feel the nurse does not understand and he may become more discouraged, hopeless, and desperate, as in the next example.

> The patient and the nurse were walking on the hospital grounds near the swimming pond. The patient began to ask the nurse questions about whether or not she could save her if she jumped into the pond. The nurse answered that she had a life-saving certificate from the Red Cross and thought she would be able to do so. The walk and such talk continued. The nurse became increasingly uncomfortable, but the patient continued to discuss the matter without apparent tension. As they approached the pond the patient jumped in and asked the nurse in a teasing, playful manner to jump in and save her. The patient swam around, dove and came up again, all the time teasing the nurse about coming in after her. The nurse sat on the bank, deciding that she wasn't going into the pond unless the patient got into difficulty. She told the patient that when she finished swimming around they'd go back for dry clothes. After awhile the patient got out and they went back to the hospital building. That evening the patient made a suicidal attempt that almost succeeded.

In thinking about the incident in retrospect, the nurse felt that the patient was trying to let her know how she felt. Because it was done in such a playful manner, she did not consider it seriously. Although she noticed her discomfort with the patient's behavior, she later felt that she had not paid close enough attention to her own reactions. She thought that the patient was trying to see if she would take her seriously and would hear her plea; when she did not, the patient "gave up" and attempted suicide.

Handling Suicidal Risks

Once the nurse has recognized that the patient is thinking about suicide and has become alerted to his tendencies or intentions, what can she do about it? What can be done to relate with the patient effectively and appropriately so as to assure his continued survival, to prevent a suicidal attempt, and to help the patient come to feel that continuation of his life is necessary and desirable?

A central problem in dealing with a suicidal patient therapeutically is one of balance—balance between therapeutic care and concern for the patient and protection of him against himself; that is, between trusting him with some freedom and ensuring that he does not hurt himself. One major task the nurse faces is to attain a delicate equilibrium in her relations with the patient in which he cannot hurt himself because of the precautions she has taken for him, while at the same time, because of what she does with him, she helps him develop the conscious idea and unconscious feeling that he does not want to take his life.

The attitudes the nurse has toward the patient and the actions she undertakes with him depend, in part, on her evaluation of how much of a risk she considers him to be at a particular time. She must make some evaluation of how great a risk the patient is, yet in many instances this is a difficult question to answer. The balance to be established here is between overestimating the risk and becoming alarmed and unnecessarily restrictive, and underestimating it and thereby giving the patient the opportunity to hurt himself. On the one hand, the nurse can ask herself whether she is inclined to overlook or dismiss as unimportant the indications the patient gives that he is thinking about killing himself. If, on the other hand, she does designate the patient a suicidal risk, she can try to determine her reasons for doing so. Does she call the patient a suicidal risk as a rationalization or excuse for imposing prohibitions and limitations that would make it convenient and justifiable for her to deal with him in a routine, impersonal, and restrictive way? It is important for the nurse to try to find out whether she is calling the patient a suicidal risk primarily for her own convenience, because of her own needs and anxiety, or whether her concern is primarily with the patient's needs and his welfare.

We indicated previously that the suicidal patient wants someone to help him, really to care for him, to be concerned about his welfare, and to think him worthwhile. Especially, he wants the nurse to *want him to live*. He also wants to be protected from himself and his possible impulsive behavior. Because the patient is not able to ask for help or to express his needs openly, the nurse must not assume that he does not want and need this help. He needs it desperately and often asks indirectly to be protected from himself. The healthy part of him wants to continue living. In order to show that she does care about his continued survival, the nurse must take seriously each suicidal threat, gesture, or indication the patient makes. Taking these threats seriously does not mean that the nurse has to become alarmed or frantic about the patient. Rather, it means that she gives the patient her attention immediately; she shows him sympathetic and serious concern; by putting herself out for the patient she shows that he really matters to her; she persists in her support of him, increases her careful observations of him, does as much as she can to reassure him and to indicate that she will do her utmost to assure his survival. In the example that follows a student nurse tells the instructor about her experiences with a patient who had made a number of attempts to injure herself. It illustrates one way in which a nurse might take the patient's threats seriously and show her concern for the patient.

MISS BALES: I don't know where Miss Smith gets hold of all the glass, but she does. We're pretty wise to it and we can tell when she has it.

INSTRUCTOR: How did you know she had glass?

MISS BALES: Well, watching her you could see that she was restless. Then when you got around her you could see that she felt guilty or you would feel that she was just trying to hide something from you. You just felt that something was wrong, and knowing her you thought about glass the first thing. You would search her, and sometimes she would give the glass to you and sometimes you would have to take it.

INSTRUCTOR: Can you give me some examples of this—when she gave it to you and when she didn't, and what she did about it?

MISS BALES: Well, once when she gave it to me it was part of a cream pitcher, I think. She would start acting restless and I could feel something wasn't quite right. I said, "Look, Rose, I think you have glass. I want it." Then she gave it to me, and I said, "Do you have any more?" and she said, "No." She has never lied to me about it. If she says "No," I believe her. One time when the ward and another patient with whom she got along were upset, we couldn't find her. We went out on the porch and she was sitting in the corner in pajamas. She had her bathrobe all wound up in her lap. When I came up to her I said, "Rose, it's pretty cold to be out here without your robe on." She jumped. I knew right then that something was wrong. So I said, "Let me have the glass." So she just handed me the whole robe and I opened it up and there was the light bulb completely smashed, with the metal base and everything. And she had her hands clenched, so I said, "Open your hands." She wasn't going to at first, and one of the aides came out then and said, "You need some help?" I handed him the robe and told him to take the glass out, to take the whole thing to the kitchen so we'd be sure it was all there. I said, "Now, Rose, I want that piece of glass you have in your hand." She said, "No." Then I just took her by the wrist and I said, "Give it to me." She just turned it loose. I thought, "Well now she is really upset, so this means something's wrong." So I said, "Well, I guess we'd better go in the bathroom and I'll search you carefully so I won't feel uncomfortable around you the rest of the day." So I took her in and stripped her completely and looked through her shoes, the seams of her clothes, even through her hair. I said, "Come on in your room and lie on your bed and I'll stay with you a while and talk to you." And she did. She was very pale and shaky, and she hadn't said anything to me the whole time. She didn't offer any resistance at all. I talked with her a while and I still was very uncomfortable with her. I just couldn't help feeling that she had more glass. So I made her get up and I searched the bed. I just couldn't find it. I told the head nurse I thought she still had some glass. We both looked. We couldn't find it anywhere, but I just knew she had it. So in a little while she said, "I want to go to the bathroom." So I went with her. She started talking about how she resented having to be searched like this. I said, "Well, you know that when you do these things the only choice we have is to search you. I'm not going to let you hurt yourself if I can help it. If you can't give it to us we have to look for it." Then I noticed that she talked a little funny, like her mouth was real full. She had had some chewing gum in her mouth. We took that away, but she still talked as though her mouth was full. I said, "Rose, you have the glass in your mouth and I want it." She said, "I'm not going to give it to you."

INSTRUCTOR: Then you knew that it was in her mouth?

MISS BALES: Yes. She didn't say it wasn't there. She said, "I'm not going to give it to you." I said, "Well, you can give it to me—which I would prefer that you do—or I can call in someone and we can take it." She said, "I'll swallow it." I said, "Well then I can't help you. But if I can take it away from you then I'm certainly going to. I'm just not going to let this happen." So I took her back on the hall and she made a dash back to the chest there in the hall. By that time other personnel saw that something was going on. I told them she had glass in her mouth, right under her tongue. So they held her and I took it away from her. Then she wanted me to stay with her.

INSTRUCTOR: How did you know she wanted you to stay with her?

MISS BALES: I asked her if she wanted to talk about it. She shook her head [no]. I said, "Well, do you want me to go?" She said, "No, I want you to stay here." So I just sat there. We didn't do much talking about it until later on when we went to the bathroom that night.

A significant aspect of the example given above is the fact that the patient did not swallow the glass although it would have been possible for her to do so. The instructor thought that the patient had to see to what lengths the student would go to show she really cared about the patient, and how much the student would persist in her efforts to protect her from herself. When the patient was convinced of the genuineness of the student's efforts, she could discontinue her attempt at self-injury.

How can the nurse show respect for the suicidal patient, trust him, and at the same time protect him from himself? How can she contribute to raising his self-esteem and at the same time make sure that means are not available in the environment with which he can injure himself? How can she maintain therapeutic opportunities for the patient's growth and development and at the same time prevent a suicidal attempt?

On the one hand, if the nurse places exclusive emphasis on protection she might put the patient under constant surveillance, in a "suicidal room," with others presumably like himself. She can restrict his freedom of movement and have him accompanied wherever he goes. However, by protecting the patient in this way she may contribute to his becoming more desperate and more determined to kill himself. This may come about in a number of ways. When his privacy is invaded to such an extreme degree the patient's feeling that he is not worthwhile and not worthy of the trust of another person is reinforced, and he is constantly confronted with evidence that life the way he has to live it is not worth living. These are the very feelings and attitudes that were in part responsible for the development of his suicidal tendencies. In addition, the patient may interpret these extreme restrictions on his freedom as punishment and become so resentful about them that he constantly seeks an opportunity to kill himself in order to "show them"—to revenge himself in this way for the deprivation he is forced to suffer. When nursing personnel constantly confront the patient with the attitude, "you are a suicidal patient," it is extremely difficult for him to have any other attitude toward himself. If everyone around him consistently looks upon him as "suicidal," how can he believe anything else about himself? Under these severely restrictive circumstances the patient's despair, desperation, and desire to kill himself may be reinforced.

On the other hand, not taking some precautions and not making a special effort to protect the patient might mean to him that the nurse really does not care if he commits suicide. Similarly, if the nurse permits dangerous instruments, such as knives and glass, to be easily available to him, the patient may interpret this as the nurse's inviting, encouraging, or wanting him to use these instruments to hurt himself. If a suicidal patient is given "unaccompanied privileges," he may feel that "they really do not care what happens to me and they really do not understand how I feel."

Thus, the nurse's problem is to find a way of dealing appropriately with the suicidal patient. She must discover how to observe him carefully and sympathetically while at the same time not make him feel that she is hovering over him, guarding him, and keeping him under constant scrutiny. If the nurse spends a great deal of time with the patient, she must learn to do it in a way that does not make him feel she is suspicious of his every move; rather, she must have and try to convey the attitude that she is doing this because she cares about him and feels he needs her. For some patients, in some circumstances, allowing or helping the patient to express his hostile and hateful feelings verbally may reduce the necessity for putting his feelings into action and turning his destructive impulses toward himself. Encouraging the overt expression of hostility and hatred does not mean, of course, that the nurse should encourage the patient to physically attack other people. The appropriateness of the nurse's relations with the patient depends not only on the particular activity she undertakes with him but also on her attitude and approach toward him. When the nurse consistently tries to make a genuine and serious effort to find the best way of helping the patient, her interest and concern for him may be crucial in keeping him alive.

An important consideration in dealing with patients who are suicidal risks is the problem of timing. How and when does the patient move out of the category of "suicidal risk"? At what point does the nurse suggest to the doctor that the first step might be taken in gradually removing the precautions that have been taken to ensure the patient's survival. If the patient is not to be deprived indefinitely of the privileges other patients have, at some point nursing and medical staff must "take a chance" with him and see if he can take more responsibility for himself. The timing of this move depends in part upon the nurse's sensitive evaluation of the patient's readiness. If she remembers that the suicidal patient also has a healthy side that wants to live and grow, she will be constantly on the alert to bring about and develop the occasions in which this part of him can express itself. One way this might be done is for her to suggest the earliest appropriate time for the patient to be given the opportunity to expand his activities. If in the patient's relations with the nurse he has an opportunity gradually to assume responsibility for his own survival and the conduct of his own life he may develop self-respect and a desire to live more adequately and satisfyingly.

PERSONNEL REACTIONS

We indicated previously the importance of the nurse's feelings about the patient and her attitudes toward him in preventing a suicidal attempt. We will now discuss the nurse's reactions to the patient who has made an unsuccessful suicidal attempt.

When a patient has attempted suicide, the nurse may be overcome with anxiety and experience other intense feelings. When the nurse discovers the patient, she may be frightened that the patient will die, that she will be unable to do anything for him, or that she will do the "wrong thing" with him. She also may feel sorry and regretful that the patient had to take such an extreme step. After the initial shock, the nurse ordinarily will mobilize herself for some action. She quickly realizes that she has to do something specific and has to do it immediately. Her training as a nurse and her desire to save the patient will help her react almost automatically with emergency procedures for the patient. In addition, if she can focus on the patient's immediate need in the emergency situation—what specifically and concretely must be done—she will be able to reduce her anxiety and handle her feelings so that they do not impair her effectiveness. When the emergency is over she can begin to sort out her feelings and reactions.

After the emergency the nurse may become concerned about the punishment she will receive from persons in authority and the blame and criticism she will receive from her colleagues. She may become preoccupied with such questions as: How am I responsible for what the patient did? Where did I slip up? What could I have done to prevent it? What are they going to do to me if they think it is my fault? In addition, she may blame herself for the patient's suicidal attempt. She may feel that she has failed in her relationship with the patient or that she did not observe him carefully enough. The nurse can blame herself or feel that others will blame her, whether or not she is actually justified in feeling this way. Usually such self-blame and anticipated blame and punishment from the persons in authority make the nurse feel anxious and insecure. Thus, *she may need reassurance and support*. It seems to us that it is much more important to focus on what went wrong in the situation than to blame and punish someone for it. In an atmosphere of punishment and blame it is usually difficult to discover what went wrong and what might be changed to prevent a recurrence. It would be much more useful to gather and evaluate as much information as possible about the circumstances that led up to the patient's suicidal attempt. In trying to discover the reasons for the failure with a particular patient, questions such as the following can be asked: What signs and cues did the patient give that were not seen or heard? What negligence or carelessness occurred? What opportunities to help the patient were missed? What relations with the patient seem not to have been of use to him?

It is common for the nurse to feel guilty when a patient attempts suicide. Her guilt is related to the anticipation of blame from others and her wondering in what ways she is responsible for the patient's action. In order to understand and handle her guilt the nurse must develop some awareness of the extent to which she can assume responsibility for a patient in these situations. It seems to us that the nurse can assume certain responsibilities but cannot assume others. She can assume the responsibility for showing concern for the patient, trying to understand and respond to his needs, giving him as much support as possible and persisting in this support, and providing protection in his environment. But the nurse cannot assume total and unconditional responsibility for a patient's life. She shares this responsibility with her nursing colleagues and the doctors in the hospital. In addition, the patient also has some responsibility in this matter, for it is his life that is involved. Furthermore, the nurse cannot provide a completely safe environment all of the time. The patient may find ways of attempting suicide despite the utmost precautions she may have taken. It is sometimes difficult to find the best way of helping a patient to continue to live when so many of his past experiences have led him to the conclusion that life is not worth living. All the nurse can do is grapple with the problem, recognizing the limits of her responsibility. If she feels that she has done as much as she can within these limits, perhaps she can then function with reduced anxiety and in a less restricted way in trying to discover and develop the relations with the patient that will help him give up his desire to do away with himself.

If the nurse looks closely at herself, she may discover that she has mixed feelings toward the patient. In addition to feeling sorry and guilty she sometimes feels angry with the patient. Her anger may stem from the feeling that the patient has put her in the position of being open to blame and criticism. She may interpret the suicidal attempt as a hostile, unfriendly gesture toward her. The nurse may blame the patient, feel critical of him, and think that his act was deliberately designed to hurt her and that he "didn't have to do this." She may feel that this is indeed small return for her efforts with him. After she becomes aware that she is angry with the patient, the nurse may feel guilty because she knows the patient is very sick, desperately in need of care, and dependent upon her for it. She may be able to handle these negative feelings more adequately if she is aware of them, however, than if she denies them to herself when they are actually present.

The nurse may feel helpless and discouraged after a patient's suicidal attempt. If she has put much effort into helping the patient she may feel that she is unable to do anything more for him. His action may convince her that she has failed with him, and she may doubt that anything she did in the past or now does for and with him counts. The nurse can expect such discouragement to arise immediately after a patient's suicidal attempt. But she can also expect that it will disappear if she focuses her attention on the ways and means of preventing future attempts.

After the patient's suicidal attempt the nurse may be concerned about the ways in which she can initiate contact with the patient. Because she is embarrassed, feels uncomfortable, and does not know what to do with the patient, she may want to avoid him. She may wonder about the kind of conversation she can carry on with the patient: "What can I say to him? Shall I ignore his suicidal attempt or talk directly to him about it?" If the nurse avoids the patient, he may feel that his behavior has been so horrible—he is so horrible—that the nurse cannot even come near him. But handling him with "kid gloves" and treating him with exaggerated care may make him uncomfortable and resentful. Thus, the nurse has to find a way of dealing with the patient, without on the one hand denying or ignoring the fact that he has made a suicidal attempt, and on the other hand without emphasizing it or forcing the patient to think or talk about it. Discussing the kind of nursing care she will have to administer to the patient while he is recuperating may help both the patient and the nurse handle some of the awkwardness and difficulty in the situation. The nurse can try to sensitize herself to the patient's wishes and give him an opportunity to talk about the incident if he wants to do so. Some patients want to talk about their feelings, want to understand what happened, and need the nurse to help them find the answers to questions they are asking. Other patients want to say as little as possible and to forget the incident as quickly as possible. The nurse may discover an appropriate way of dealing with the patient if she keeps her focus on understanding him and forming a relationship with him in which he feels that life is worthwhile because he can find some satisfaction in it.

‹ 10 ›

The Patient Is Extremely Anxious

THE patient's anxiety will enter into many of the situations in which he participates. Anxiety is an important component of assaultiveness, incontinence, demandingness, eating difficulties, hallucinations and delusions, withdrawal, and suicidal preoccupations. When we described these situations in earlier chapters we dealt with the patient's anxiety as only one aspect of the situation. In this chapter we will focus on patient anxiety in its extreme forms: panic, agitation, and excitement. We will try to understand the type of overt behavior with which the patient expresses his extreme anxiety by examining what this behavior means to the patient, what brings it about, the reaction of personnel to it, and how a nurse might handle the patient's anxiety to reduce it and alleviate his discomfort.

Panic is probably the most extreme form of disturbed behavior. It is difficult for those of us who have not experienced panic to imagine what it is like. It is hard to imagine the dread, the terror, and the intense anguish the patient suffers. In a panic state the patient seems unaware of what is happening to him—what he is doing or what others are doing with him. He may be confused, hallucinating, raving, ranting, shouting, or screaming. His physical movements may be uncoordinated, random, explosive, or impulsive, as if he were struggling to escape some danger. At these times the tension is so great that personnel inevitably are affected by it. We cannot see such anguish, suffering, and pain without being moved—sometimes profoundly. Such important life-and-death matters are involved that it touches something vital in all of us.

Patients experience extreme anxiety in forms other than panic. When they are extremely anxious some patients become agitated, weep, moan, scream, cling to personnel, wring their hands, and pace up and down. Others are excited, talk loudly and rapidly, make quick movements, dart about in an undirected way, using as much energy as possible in the slightest activity they undertake. Still others are desperately afraid that they are going to die or be murdered, or that they will murder someone else.

How Patient Disturbances Arise

From one point of view we might say the disturbance starts "within" the patient; that is, he is "seeing things," thinking thoughts, or experiencing feelings that he cannot tolerate and that are upsetting to him. Looking at it another way, we can say that the disturbance starts "in the environment"; that is, something that happens outside the patient affects him deeply. We think a better understanding of states of extreme anxiety will develop if we can see the disturbance as a combination of internal conditions and external factors; both what is inside the patient and what affects him from the outside bring about the disturbance and maintain it.

It is very difficult to know what in the patient "sets him off" into an extremely anxious state. It may be that at that moment he recognizes something "awful" about himself; he feels threatened by some unknown force; he is disturbed by thoughts of homosexual activity; or he is afraid of being destroyed or of engaging in violence. Another possibility is that rather than particular thoughts and feelings generating the patient's disturbance, there may have been a gradual accumulation of anxiety, anxiety that is vague and difficult to specify, which has gradually grown and increased until it reaches the bursting point. For example:

> MISS ADAMS: When Carol gets into one of her upsets she begins to rage. She spits, kicks, begs for a pack, begs for you to hold onto her, and she'll throw anything she can get her hands on.
> SOCIOLOGIST: Do you have any idea what causes her upset?
> MISS ADAMS: It seems to build up for a few days. We say on the ward that Carol "is dark." Her lips are blue, her face is blue, and she

has that tense, drawn look. She really looks dark. When I first saw her this way I thought she was in a fugue state. She had no idea who you were.

MRS. BARKER: She just seems to bottle up her tension so long and then it just boils all over. She slams her door, screams, and then seems to almost disintegrate. You know what it is because the scream is the same every time.

MISS ADAMS: During her raving, she will say, "I'm so damned sick —I have been so sick—I'll never get well." She talks about what they did to her in another hospital and what they're doing to her here. Then she'll scream, "I hate you. I hate myself for being so sick."

Patients often do not know how their disturbances came about —what fantasies or feelings have stimulated their anxiety. If they know, or think they know, they frequently are unable to tell others. One of the reasons is that they feel "it's too horrible to talk about."

In addition to the patient's internal state, something in the environment may contribute to or maintain his disturbance. If the nurse is to help the patient in a disturbed state, she must try to discover what this "something" is.

There are two main factors in a patient's environment that can precipitate or contribute to his disturbance. One of these is other patients. When one patient or many patients are extremely anxious, they quickly convey this anxiety to other patients. Sometimes this communication of anxiety reaches the point where many patients are upset at the same time, continuing and reinforcing each other's disturbance. The other factor is the personnel. We have found that patients become upset when staff members are themselves extremely anxious, upset, in conflict with each other, or when they are discouraged or uncertain about what they are doing. Because personnel are so important to patients and because they are in continuous contact with them, patients are adversely affected by manifestations of serious disturbance and insecurity on the staff's part, and by continuing conflict and disagreement among personnel. Thus, one of the important things nurses can do is to become aware of the kinds of relations they carry on among themselves that are anxiety-provoking for patients.

PERSONNEL REACTIONS

Regardless of how or where the patient's upset starts, it is important for the nurse to recognize that she can play a significant part in maintaining, increasing, or reducing it. In order to become effective in reducing the patient's disturbance, the nurse has to become aware of her own reactions during these periods and of how her feelings impel her to undertake certain activities. For example, a frequent impulse of the nurse is to seclude the extremely anxious patient, removing him from others as well as from herself. She may want to escape from the situation and let someone else handle it. She may become petrified while the patient is extremely upset, or she may be at a loss to know what to do for him. In each of these instances the patient's disturbance arouses anxiety, uneasiness, or emotional disturbance in her. At times the nurse's feelings may incapacitate her temporarily, and she may become so upset that she has to escape from the patient.

> MISS TERRY: In the morning Zelda was terrified. In the afternoon she became so upset it was pitiful. She was banging on the floor screaming, "I'm being tortured; why is she torturing me so?" I was afraid to go in because in the morning she had attacked someone who went into her room. I was in a turmoil; I wanted to help her but I was frightened. Two of us opened her door and went in. As soon as we came in she said, "Come in, I won't hurt you." She said it in an imploring way and I guess she must have seen how hesitant we were. She grabbed my hand and wept bitterly. She said she was being tortured, and raved and ranted that she was going to sear "that woman" with fire and cut her into little pieces. While I sat with her my heart was torn. I couldn't stay with her. I had to go into the kitchen and cry.

In the illustration above the nurse is so vulnerable to the patient's disturbance that she is made ineffective. Once the nurse is aware of her vulnerability to the patient's extreme anxiety, she has to discover ways of dealing with her own distress so that she can be of help to the patient.

At times a patient's agitated behavior may provoke anger, annoyance, or impatience in the nurse—especially if the disturbed behavior is directed specifically toward her. Recognizing these feelings may help the nurse handle them and also help her deal usefully with the patient.

> Miss Coombs: Miss Smith makes me so angry sometimes with her hysterical crying and screaming. I was doing my best to help her and she kept screaming at me.
>
> Sociologist: If you watch your feelings as you go along, you'll learn to handle them. Once you can get your own feelings straightened out, then maybe you can help her. By getting angry or annoyed, you're more ineffective. You can't help this, but it is important that you see these feelings in yourself. When I went in to see her she also made me mad. As soon as I recognized how mad I was I felt a little better. I was able to say in a calm voice, "Miss Smith, if you're going to continue to scream and cry while I'm here, I won't be able to do you any good." She quieted down a little bit. But you have to have confidence that you can become aware of what's going on inside you. Otherwise you're battling with your own feelings and these feelings get in your way, and you don't have much control over what you can do.

The nurse's attempts to protect herself against the patient's disturbance are most subtle and difficult to become aware of. She may act as if the patient is not disturbed or is not there. She may become severely restricted in her focus, not hearing the patient's screams nor seeing his disturbed actions, not because she is deliberately ignoring them but because she is unconsciously blocking them out and is genuinely unaware of them. Obviously, it is impossible to alleviate the patient's extreme anxiety if the nurse is unaware of it. However, nurses are usually very much aware of a patient's disturbance, struggle with their reactions toward it, and try to develop more recognition of what these reactions consist of and how best to handle them. In the ways suggested above nurses try to protect themselves against the full emotional impact of the patient's disturbance.

Handling Patients' Extreme Anxiety

Discovering effective ways of handling situations in which patients show extreme anxiety is a difficult and challenging task for the nurse. It is also an extremely vital one because a patient in a panic or agitated state can die of exhaustion if he continues his extremely anxious behavior for a long period of time. Effective handling of the patient's disturbance depends, in part, on the nurse's general understanding of the sources and nature of the disturbance, on her own reactions to the disturbance itself, and on her experience and knowledge in handling patients when they are extremely upset.

One of the things a nurse can do is to try to anticipate and prevent a patient's mild disturbance from developing into an extreme one. If the nurse knows the patient well, she may be able to identify early signs of disturbance. These signs may be revealed in the patient's face, in the way he moves, in the kinds of gestures he makes, in the content and form of his talk, and in the kinds of stereotyped activity he performs. If the nurse is alert to early signs of patient disturbance, she may be able to alleviate the patient's anxiety with much less effort and more effectively than if she waits until his disturbance has increased.

> MRS. DIAMOND: I've learned from experience with Miss Corbett that if you don't stop her at the beginning of her upset, she gets worse. She was out on the porch very tense, and instead of taking her into the room, two of the aides just stood by her. She became more upset. Pretty soon she was screeching, and when we tried to seclude her she struggled violently. It took three of us to handle her.
>
> MISS BECKER: Sometimes when she's beginning to get excited, I've talked with her a few minutes and that has calmed her. She responds to someone's interest in her when she's upset. I think she wants you to be with her when she starts blowing up.

If these early signs of upset are ignored or not recognized, the patient may become increasingly anxious, and his disturbance may contribute to a more generalized disturbance among other patients.

> HEAD NURSE: Betty became upset and started yelling this morning. She kept getting higher and higher. Doris was standing around, and she started getting upset. So the first mistake we made was not getting Betty into her room right away instead of letting her continue to yell in the hall. Ann began shaking her finger in her excited way and nobody went over to her. Soon she was shaking her finger at Zelda, and Zelda blew up. She went into her room, slammed the

door a few times, and shouted at her roommate to get out and then threw her out. Nobody went in with Zelda to try and quiet her. In the midst of all this, Rose started leaping up and down, cussing, talking about filthy animals, and screaming at the top of her lungs. Both Miss Jones and Miss Jackson [two nurses] were just petrified; they didn't make a move. Finally, I took Rose to her room. By this time Claire had become upset and was raving about systems of persecution.

SOCIOLOGIST: The important thing is to do something about the situation when you see it beginning to build up. The more it builds up the more difficult it is to keep it in check. If you get into it as close to the beginning as possible, you have a much better chance of preventing the upset from spreading. I would have tried to give each patient individual attention with whatever staff you had, and I would have tried to separate them from each other. You could keep them away from each other by seclusion and by taking one patient to another part of the ward.

When the nurse is not able to anticipate and prevent a patient's upset, she can try to work out a way of dealing with him in his disturbed state. *What the patient needs most in these situations is reassurance*—reassurance that reaches him, is persistent, is acceptable to him, is appropriate for him, and is experienced as genuine by him. The patient is desperate for someone's help, for someone to convey to him that he or his situation is not so horrible as he thinks. In trying to alleviate his desperate state, pity or condescension or a stereotyped, routine, or impersonal response is not likely to be of much help. The reassurance the patient needs can take many forms and must be given differently to different patients if it is to be effective. In order to give this reassurance it is not necessary for the nurse to understand what the patient thinks is disturbing him, nor to clarify for him the causes of his disturbance. Sometimes the nurse *does not have to do anything;* just sitting with the patient or holding his hand without saying a word may be reassuring. This may be true especially if the nurse and patient have had a good relationship previously.

As is illustrated below, the patient can accept reassurance more easily from a person she knows and with whom in the past she has had friendly experiences; the nurse can respond more freely and appropriately to a patient with whom she is familiar and toward whom she has warm feelings.

MISS ADAMS: Marjorie went into a panic state this afternoon, and I stayed with her awhile because I have discovered that sitting with her helps. Most of the time I can't get through to her, but I'm there and she knows it.

SOCIOLOGIST: I wouldn't worry too much about getting through. The fact that you are there is important. Can you hold her or put your arms around her?

MISS ADAMS: Sometimes I can, but today I couldn't. She wouldn't let me.

SOCIOLOGIST: Maybe all you can do is have a quiet, accepting attitude without saying anything. At these times it doesn't make any sense to try and reason with her.

MISS ADAMS: She knew I was there. She called out my name. I think what's important, too, is that we have a good relationship. When she gets into a panic state I can handle it better than someone she doesn't know very well or who hasn't had much experience with her.

SOCIOLOGIST: I think it might be useful to notice the things in the situation that give her some relief or help her out of the panic.

MISS ADAMS: The important thing is to treat the panic as an emergency situation and try to give her as much attention and nursing care as possible.

Sometimes, if her reassurance is to be effective with the patient, the nurse may have to be a little more active than "just being with the patient."

MISS BECKER: Joan blew up today. She started to scream and yell, throwing her hands and feet around. Helen Jackson [a nurse] came over, took Joan's hands, and sat down on the bed with her. Joan kept screaming about being raped and about babies. She told Miss Jackson to get out, but Miss Jackson said, "I'm going to stay with you." Joan screamed for about fifteen minutes. Helen held her hands for some time and kept repeating, "Don't you know me, Joan? I'm Miss Jackson, a nurse." At first Joan said, "No," to her questions, but after a while she relaxed and quieted down. Helen sat with her twenty minutes, washed her face, and tucked her into bed.

In order to be reassuring to an upset patient the nurse might have to withstand rejection, threats, or assault. If despite these she can persist in her attempts to reassure the patient, she may find that the patient accepts her and benefits from her reassurance.

> MISS ALLEN: You know Alice is the kind of patient who gets very assaultive when she's upset. She's supposed to be able to really hurt you. We were told not to go near her when she became upset. I thought I'd try to see what would happen if I did stay with her. I followed her into her room, and she said, "Get out." I said I wasn't leaving, that I would stay with her. I sat with her in the room, and she quieted down soon. One time she turned to me and said, "You know how sick I am," and she held onto my arms.

In order to reassure the patient the nurse may have to withstand much anguish herself and spend a considerable amount of time with the patient while the latter is enduring indescribable agony.

> MISS CRESSY: She began screaming, "Criminals, murderers," and crying, "I can't stand it! I can't stand it!" First I said, "What can't you stand?" but this was only confusing to her. So I just said, "I will stay with you," and she finally got so that she was holding onto me for dear life. When she grabbed me, she looked as terrified as I have ever seen a patient. It was really terrible panic, and she started moaning and groaning, "It's horrible, it's horrible!" I kept thinking to myself how much she was going through. She kept yelling at me, "Do something! Can't you do something? Can't you see I'm in agony?" All I said was, "I guess you have to go through this, but I will stay with you." All of a sudden she was incontinent, so I got her out of bed. She looked at the urine as if it were blood, and she was just terrified. She was just raving. A student came in, and it took two of us to hold her. She would push up against us, then pull away, then she would grab me, then grab the student. She didn't know what she was doing. We changed her bed and got her back into bed and covered her up. Then she started shaking, so we got some ice water and some milk, and I gave her small sips. After this she quieted down.

In some situations patients are so desperate that they will beg the nurse to calm the terror they feel.

> MR. HOLDEN: Mary was very disturbed about something; she clung to me and begged me to stay with her awhile. She clutched my hand and kept repeating, "Please stay with me." She was just scared to death and she wanted someone near her. I know if I were as frightened, I would, too.

If the patient does not get the reassurance he needs, if it is given to him in a way that he cannot accept, or if it does not reach him, his disturbance may grow to terrifying proportions. In these situations the patient is in danger of exhausting or physically injuring himself, and at the same time he strains the nurse's endurance, imagination, and ability to give him reassurance. In the example that follows we see how a nurse was helpful to an extremely agitated patient who was wearing herself out and assaulting herself.

MISS ALLEN: Carrie has been pulling out her hair, beating herself, and pacing back and forth on the ward. We've been packing her to prevent the hair pulling, and I've been pacing with her to try to quiet her. When we took her to her room she started beating herself on the door. The more I'd try to stop her the more she'd beat herself. We tried to get her undressed to pack her, but she went out in the hall and started pacing. I paced with her and took off her clothes one piece at a time until she was in her slip, and then we took her into her room and packed her. The pack seems to help, but out of it she hits herself all the time. We try physically to prevent her from doing this. Sometimes I hold her hands. When she paces in this agitated way I put my arms around her and walk with her. I've even fed some patients like her while pacing with them. But as soon as I leave Carrie alone she starts hurting herself again.

When she's not grabbing onto us she's pacing. She keeps saying, "Take me home! Let me die!" About all we can do with her is pace up and down with her and see that she drinks enough. We keep taking her water and fruit juice. I put my arm around her and walk up and down with her while she drinks it.

MISS BROOME: How can we step in and prevent her from exhausting herself?

MISS ALLEN: She's in pack about six hours a day, but they don't do much good. Last night she was pacing and I grabbed her when she went past her room and said, "You're coming in here with me and you're going to lie down on your bed and rest." She did lie down. I covered her up and she rested for about half an hour. I stayed with her while she rested.

MISS BROOME: How come that worked?

MISS ALLEN: I'll never know.

MISS BROOME: Maybe it worked because you were firm. I remember a patient like Carrie. I'd get her into bed, and the only way to keep her in bed was to go through the motions of doing things. We made believe we were running a race with our fingers.

MISS ALLEN: Pacing helps with patients like her. Also, I used to get agitated patients to tear rags and wind them into balls. Giving them something to scrub or to sweep also seemed to help, especially if you did it with them.

Several days later there was another discussion about this patient.

MISS ALLEN: I sat her on the chair and started rocking her back and forth, and that really did the trick. Some of the others took over and rocked her all evening, and she didn't pace, nor did she pace the next day.

MISS BROOME: How did you happen to think of rocking her?

MISS ALLEN: I had been pacing with her, and I just led her to the chair, thinking maybe she'd sit in it. She started getting up out of the chair and I put my arm in front of her and rocked the chair back and forth, and she just relaxed.

In the illustration above the nurse had to strain her imagination to discover ways to reassure the patient, but she was able to find some that were useful. Apparently her persistence reached the patient. In addition the patient may have been responding to the nurse's interest and concern for her as evidenced by her strenuous efforts to help.

In the example that follows an aide was reassuring to a patient who manifested her anxiety by screaming and clinging to personnel during her upsets. Because of this behavior, personnel became rejecting of her. The aide, however, was effective because she was both definite in her instructions to the patient and persisted in her attempts to clarify her statements to her.

SOCIOLOGIST: Can you tell me what you do with Miss Smith that is helpful to her?

MRS. BYERS: When she gets upset I go in very quietly. I don't get so involved that I can't tolerate her.

SOCIOLOGIST: Doesn't she make you anxious when she gets into that screaming state?

MRS. BYERS: No.

SOCIOLOGIST: What does she make you feel?

MRS. BYERS: She makes me feel like a mother. I want to hold her and say, "Let's weather this storm together and everything will be all right." One day she was very upset and was pacing up and down. She was going around in circles and said she was dizzy. I said, "I know you are, and you'll get dizzier if you keep walking that way. Now you lie down and rest until the dizziness passes." She dozed for about a half hour. I sat with her and she woke up and said, "Can I get up now?" I said, "No, lie down and rest," and she'd rest awhile.

SOCIOLOGIST: How would you account for the fact that you've been so effective in handling her?

MRS. BYERS: I don't know. I've learned patience with her. I've looked upon it as a challenge. With anyone as upset as Miss Smith, I don't think it makes much difference what you say, but if you say it simply and over and over again it will finally sink in, especially if you say it each time in the same way.

One obvious aspect of these situations in which the patient is extremely anxious is that the patient cannot control his behavior. The patient's anxiety will not disappear suddenly, nor will he stop behaving in an upset way if he tells himself or the nurse says, "Stop being upset." There are times, however, when the patient can use the help he gets from the nurse's telling him to stop some particular kind of behavior. Stopping the particular behavior might reduce the patient's upset slightly, even though on the whole he still is extremely anxious. At these times it may be that the nurse is reassuring to the patient—at least temporarily— when she indicates to him that *she thinks he can stop*. This may be true especially for a patient who believes he is not able to do anything at all about his behavior, that it is outside of his control. The patient can be reassured by the nurse's attitude that he is not completely powerless in the situation, and with her help can feel he is doing something about his behavior.

MISS CRANE: Yesterday Miss Jones was packed because she was upset. When I went in with her tube-feeding she got more upset. Finally, after she'd been shaking I just said to her, "Stop, Miss Jones." She said, "I can't." Then I said, "Yes, you can. You're making yourself shake." She looked at me a minute and then stopped. She stopped for about fifteen minutes and then started again. Also she began to scream and cry. I said, "Miss Jones, you aren't crying." And she said, "I'm not?" I said, "No, you don't have any tears in your eyes." She sat there for a few minutes quietly and then said, "Well, maybe I don't have any tears left; maybe I'm not capable of crying any more." When I would tell her to stop what she was doing, she would become very relaxed, almost as if she were asleep. Also, each time that I told her something directly she would relax. At one point she kept screaming at me until I couldn't take it any longer. I said, "Stop screaming at me." She stopped and said, "I'm not screaming at you." I said, "You were." She then would talk in a very low voice for a while.

Some excited patients need the security of a definite routine. A patient may be reassured if the nurse can tell him what his activities will be during the day. Taking the patient in on planning for his own care sometimes helps.

HEAD NURSE: Today we were really desperate about Joan. We spent the whole morning figuring out what we were going to do with her. She was walking up and down the halls shouting, going out on the porch and yelling at everybody on the grounds. We tried giving her a pack. That didn't work. We gave her some sedation and she got "high" on that. We had people specialing her continuously, but she wore them out. No one could stand her long, so we went on shifts. We posted a schedule and there was a change every forty-five minutes. That turned out to be too stimulating for her—so many different people. But one person just couldn't stand her for more than a short time. We finally called her into the office and told her we were at the end of our rope. "What would you suggest we do to help you quiet down?" We didn't decide anything, but after that she quieted down.

The next day we decided that giving her a schedule might help. We planned all the things she would do during the day—when she would be secluded, when specialed, when she could be out on the hall. We also told her we'd seclude her if she became noisy on the hall. The schedule seemed to help her because she was fairly quiet.

There are times when the nurse has to do something about the patient's environment in order to give him reassurance. Sometimes a patient has to be removed from other patients because constant contact with others continues or increases his disturbance. One head nurse found it useful to seclude for long periods a patient who became increasingly upset each time she came out of her room. She had a staff member go in and stay with the patient part of the time. In such a situation it is important for the staff member to be able to withstand the patient's anxiety and for her to want to stay with the patient in seclusion. If she feels "put upon," she is not likely to be helpful to the patient.

In reducing a patient's contacts with others in order to help him become less disturbed, it is important in most instances not to leave the patient completely alone. But occasionally the patient may calm down when left alone. The nurse should watch carefully to see if the patient is actually helped by being left alone; she should return frequently to find out whether he gives any indication of wanting or being able to use her company. In most of these crisis situations it seems to us that the patient desperately needs the nurse. All alone with his immense anxiety, he may feel utterly abandoned. The comfort and reassurance he gets from the nurse's presence may be of considerable significance to him—especially the fact that she accepts him during his upset state. Therefore, when she decides to seclude an upset patient, it is important that she be sure that she is not doing this just for her own convenience.

A patient in a disturbed state may sometimes be helped by prompt and definite action on the nurse's part. The patient may be reassured if the nurse knows what she is doing and does it effectively. One way of establishing favorable conditions for effective operation by the nurse is to work out smoothly functioning team activity among staff members to deal with the patient when he becomes upset and to see the upset through with him. One aspect of this teamwork is getting the staff members to agree on the procedure to be used with a disturbed patient and on what each of the personnel will do in the immediate situation when a patient is extremely anxious and more than one person is needed to deal with him. By working together effectively staff members develop a sense of security in handling the patient, and when the security of the staff is experienced by the patient, it may be reassuring to him.

Sometimes the nurse may mistake a patient's agitated or excited behavior as an attack upon her and react to it with fear. It is important for the nurse to recognize how desperately the patient needs her help in such a situation, so that she is not driven away by his seemingly threatening behavior. It may often seem to the nurse who is in a situation with an extremely disturbed patient that it is almost impossible to discover what can help him. Ordinarily she does not know ahead of time what will help each patient. On the basis of past experiences she may know a few effective measures. In the examples we have given, and from our observations, what seems to be important is the nurse's feeling that she could discover some way to be helpful if she looked long enough and carefully enough. It is important for the nurse to be willing to put forth much energy and thought, that is, "put herself out" in order to reassure the patient, because his disturbance is of serious concern to her. The nurse's willingness and ability to withstand her own anxiety, as well as other unpleasant feelings and difficulties in order to try to reduce the patient's anxiety, is of utmost importance in helping the extremely anxious patient.

Summary

At this point it might be helpful to summarize the general ideas we have set forth in our discussion of problem situations and to show their implications for relations with patients.

When a patient develops a pattern of difficulty such as incontinence, assaultiveness, withdrawal, and so on, the nurse is confronted with a problem situation which she tries to solve. The interpersonal relations she carries on in general with the patient and those she maintains specifically with reference to his pattern of difficulty can either help to sustain and reinforce the patient's behavior or contribute to changing and eliminating it.

In a problem situation, the patient relates to the nurse with his pattern of difficulty and the nurse responds to it. The patient, in turn, responds to her response, and this, again, elicits another reaction from the nurse. Thus, there is continuing interaction—action and reaction, response and counterresponse—between the patient and the nurse. Through this interaction each contributes to making the relationship what it is and what it will become. In this chain of interaction the nurse affects the patient in many ways, and the patient also influences the nurse. Because of the reciprocal influences the patient and nurse have on each other, they can modify or reinforce each other's behavior in significant ways. The nurse's therapeutic task is to observe and to develop a clearer awareness of the subtleties in her relations with the patient. With this awareness she can try to change her responses to the patient so that the patient will be able to change his responses to her; she can try to maintain their relations with each other in such a way that the patient will no longer find it necessary to continue his pattern of difficulty. This does not mean that the nurse forces the patient to change but that the change in his behavior emerges from their relationship; that is to say, the patient changes because of the way he and the nurse are participating together.

This view of mutual participation has a number of aspects. The patient is not just a passive recipient of the nurse's care, nor is he an object to be moved around by her. He is an active participant in the relationship, and his activity has important effects on it. The patient is not impervious to the nurse's attitudes toward him and her activities with him. It is not only that the nurse *"does something for and with"* the patient, but the patient *"does something to and with"* her and for himself. Because the patient is mentally ill, the nurse must be ready to take the initiative in encouraging his participation and in taking him in as an active partner in their relationship. She tries to work with him toward the fulfillment of his needs so that therapeutic benefit will emerge for the patient. This does not mean that the nurse "takes over" without finding out what the patient's desires are. It means, rather, that to the degree that he is able, the nurse enlists the patient's participation in making decisions about his own care. It also means that the responsibility for the maintenance of the patient's patterns of difficulty is shared by both patient and nurse and others, as is the responsibility for improvement in his mental health.

In discussing these problem situations we have selected only some that are commonly met by nurses. There are, of course, others. We believe that the approach we have used in understanding the interpersonal relations between nurse and patient in these situations is applicable to the types of problem situations a nurse meets on a mental hospital ward. In addition, when we have discussed the patient's participation in these problem situations, referring to him as a withdrawn patient, an assaultive patient, and so on, we have focused on only one aspect of the patient. We have made this selection not on the basis of the patient's diagnostic classification, but in terms of one dominant type of behavior that is troublesome for him and at the same time is a problem that the nurse must handle. We would like to emphasize, however, that the patient is more than just this selected aspect—more, for example, than an assaultive or autistic patient. He has the potentiality for other ways of behaving and he actually engages in many different types of behavior in any one day. Thus, the "patient as a whole"—with all the various aspects of his behavior—must be considered in evaluating and dealing with any problem situation.

It is also important to emphasize that in responding to the patient or in trying to deal with him the nurse should avoid using a technique—a preestablished, calculated procedure for relating with him—or a pat formula as a way of approaching him. We would suggest that the nurse not plan precisely what she is going to do and say with the patient nor think in terms of manipulating him. Rather, we suggest that the helpful, appropriate response can be discovered in the situation itself—can be discovered while the nurse is carrying on interpersonal activity with the patient. If the nurse can permit herself to be spontaneous in her relations with the patient, she may discover that her warmth toward him and her understanding of him grow. If her awareness of herself and the patient expands and her perspective on the situation broadens, her responses and activities may bring about a satisfying experience for the patient and contribute to the resolution of the problem situation.

We also wish to point out the importance of the time factor in these problem situations. A patient repeatedly may present the same problem to the nurse. If the problem situation is to be resolved, the nurse may have to persist in her efforts with the patient over a long period of time. In the course of her continuing experience with the patient, the nurse has an opportunity to learn and to grow. Her awareness and skill may develop at the same time that the patient acquires greater trust in her. This increasing familiarity and this trust might contribute to the gradual alleviation and elimination of the problem situation and to the facilitation of the patient's mental health.

PART II

INTERPERSONAL PROCESSES COMMON
TO PROBLEM SITUATIONS

‹ 11 ›

The Nurse and the Patient—
An Illustration

IN Part I we discussed a number of problem situations, focusing
on the ways in which the nurse and patient affect each other.
In Part II we will discuss interpersonal processes that are common to these situations. In order to deal effectively with each
type of situation the nurse tries to understand the patient and
tries to communicate with and relate to him in a way that will be
mutually satisfying.

To illustrate some aspects of the subject matter that will be
discussed in this section we present an example of a nurse's participation with a patient that was meaningful and useful to both.
This example indicates the variety and complexity of elements
that enter into a nurse-patient relationship if it continues over a
period of time. In addition, it illustrates in a more comprehensive
way the kind of nursing approach we have been describing in
earlier chapters.

John Cooper was a man in his midthirties who had been in and
out of mental hospitals since early childhood. His appearance and
behavior were bizarre: he twitched, grimaced, and drooled, with
his mouth often crammed with food. His posture was twisted and
rigid, and his stooped body jerked when he walked. Sometimes
he shook as if he were very frightened. His infrequent attempts to
speak usually resulted only in grunts and groans, but he managed
to say a few words when he wanted something badly. Mr. Cooper
had many crying spells and had childlike temper tantrums in
which he lay on the floor screaming and kicking. At other times

he would reach for the arm or the skirt of a nurse passing by and cling desperately to her.

The patient refused to let food or drink be taken from him even though he had kept it for hours. He ate with both hands, getting food in his hair and ears. He clutched at his own food, took it to bed with him, and grabbed at the remains on other patients' trays. Almost constantly one hand held a cup of fruit juice, coffee, or water in a precarious position. He gave the impression of being in fear that he would die of hunger and thirst.

Personnel often had a difficult time dealing with Mr. Cooper. They tended to shrink from any physical contact with him and sometimes expressed feelings of disgust. There was talk of excluding him from patient social functions.

At one point during Mr. Cooper's stay on the ward a new aide, Ruth Lamson, came to work there. This was her first job in psychiatric nursing. The first time she appeared on the ward Mr. Cooper singled her out and attached himself to her. Within a week he was following her, putting his arms around her, clinging to her, and occasionally trying to kiss her. This behavior was embarrassing to the aide, and her discomfort increased when the personnel made remarks such as, "Are you aware of John's grand passion for Ruth?"

Miss Lamson felt sufficiently interested in the patient and uncomfortable about the situation to discuss it with the head nurse. On hearing the details, instead of reproaching her as Ruth half expected, the head nurse said, "I think this is very good. This is a valuable experience for him if you can only carry it further. Here is a man who is half dead to the world, and you awaken his interest, even if he shows it in this exaggerated way. You can't expect him to approach you as anybody else would. What can we do to use his approaches to you in a constructive way? If the staff discourages you or you become too anxious and rebuff him, the relationship will be cut off and the patient will crawl back into his shell."

The head nurse discussed the situation with a supervisor, who remarked, "It sounds to me as if Ruth is doing well with the patient and that there are potentialities for a constructive relationship. She gets embarrassed by John's falling all over her, but it would seem as though she is handling the situation well. I think the problem is to help her recognize that he needs some affection and help her give it to him."

It was clear to the doctor in charge of the ward, the head nurse, and the sociologist that John was reaching out for a relationship but that Ruth was not comfortable about his behavior. The head nurse suggested to Ruth that they discuss the situation at the weekly ward staff meeting. Ruth eagerly agreed to this.

DR. HUGHES: We have the feeling that John's interest in you represents more mature behavior on his part. We thought by talking with you we might see how we could be of assistance to you in helping him progress to possibly even a higher level of participation.

RUTH: I'd like a little direction. My whole activity with him has been so negative that I don't see how I could be doing anything for him. People say that he is responding, but I just don't know what it is that I'm doing that is helpful to him. Every time he follows me around, or tries to squeeze me, all I do is push him away and start lecturing him. I say, "You shouldn't do this and you shouldn't do that, and you know by now that you shouldn't do this." I just feel that there are some more positive things I could be doing. It seems to be a good relationship, but I don't know why.

SOCIOLOGIST: Why are you so uncomfortable about what he does that you have to lecture him?

RUTH: Well, he comes and puts his arm around me and tries to kiss me, or he even kneels down by me if I'm sitting and starts to touch me.

SOCIOLOGIST: You mean you don't like to have a man make passes at you?

RUTH: Well, he embarrasses me in front of all those people! He causes a scene. It is very unpleasant for me and for the other members of the group.

HEAD NURSE: Now my feeling is that this is putting Ruth on the spot. Still, John's behavior with her is a lot more mature than it has been with anyone else. I think he wants a relationship with Ruth and a little affection rather than a sexual exchange. But I'm sure most people on the ward interpret this as a sexual approach, and Ruth is put in an embarrassing position. I've heard a lot of kidding remarks about it.

SOCIOLOGIST: I think it's interesting and worthwhile to explore why you get so uncomfortable. I think you may have some feeling about what other personnel think.

RUTH: Sure, that's true.

SOCIOLOGIST: If we can get this straightened out—if we can understand that this is very important for John—maybe we can be helpful to him by helping Ruth relate to him. Maybe Ruth can develop some genuine concern and real affection for him. Maybe this is being blocked, in part, by the attitudes the other personnel are taking toward it.

RUTH: I have initiated very few contacts myself with John.

SOCIOLOGIST: Because you wanted to avoid him?

RUTH: Yes. Another thing—I wondered if I should try to get out of this situation, that is, run away from it, or should I try to work it out with him.

SOCIOLOGIST: You might want to settle it for yourself, but that would not necessarily mean any benefit to John. You might be able to discourage him from doing things that embarrass you, but you would not be helping him any. Edna, would you tell us how you would handle the situation or suggest how Ruth should handle it? What did you do with George Spence when he behaved somewhat like John?

EDNA: I responded by putting my arm around him, giving him a hug, and patting him on the back.

RUTH: Well, I would feel very self-conscious about hugging John.

EDNA: I did, too, at the beginning.

SOCIOLOGIST: The point is that if you make a sexual interpretation of his activity, you're going to be uncomfortable. But if you can see John as somebody who needs a little warmth, a little affection, somewhat like a small child, and also that his activity has other elements in it, then I think it will be easier to put your arm around him or pat him on the back.

RUTH: But I don't like to treat him like a child, because obviously he is not a child.

SOCIOLOGIST: But this is the kind of warmth John wants. I don't think you are being contemptuous of him or treating him like a child when you try to give him what he wants and needs. Your respect for him will come out in the way you give him this affection. It seems to me he needs this kind of warmth at this time—to feel that someone can touch him and he can feel comforted by it.

HEAD NURSE: I think if you would go to him instead of his always having to run after you, that would help. Also, if you would spend some time with him because you wanted to do so. I think he is looking for some attention from you. He is looking for someone to be friendly with, and if you give him this friendship he might stop falling all over you.

SOCIOLOGIST: If somebody does something unpleasant to you and if you have confidence in that person, you'll try to talk with him about it and get it straightened out. Well, why not with John? Why not tell him you'd like to be friends with him and that he doesn't have to hang onto you?

DR. HUGHES: After all, the big problem with many patients is that they are so passive about trying to get their needs fulfilled that we have to worry about what it is they want and how to do it for them. But this man is really doing something about it. I think that's quite important.

RUTH: Well, I think I've picked up a few pretty good points. I think I'll see him and talk to him. I doubt if I'll get much in the way of a two-way conversation, but at least I will talk to him, and one of the things I might mention is that we can be friends without that other stuff.

When Ruth returned to the ward she did not wait for John to come to her but went immediately to talk with him. She told John that she would like to be friends with him, and that it was not necessary for him to cling to her; she would spend time with him when she could. She also told John she was interested in him and liked him. While she talked with him she patted him on the back. The patient seemed pleased and seemed to accept what Ruth said. As a matter of fact, after this talk John no longer clung to her or embarrassed her by the behavior discussed at the conference.

Ruth talked with the head nurse about John's reactions, and while discussing the patient recalled her own reactions the first time John had tried to kiss her.

RUTH: It came as a shock to me because I didn't expect this behavior from him. I had never considered him *that human*. I realized then that he was a person with the same feelings as anyone else. That was the first time I really saw him as a person.

HEAD NURSE: What do you mean when you say you began to see him as a person?

RUTH: The first time I saw John I thought he was an old man. He had on an old coat and he wasn't shaved. He was all huddled up, with no collar, hair not combed. I remember thinking, "He is probably about fifty years old, not an old man but getting on"—a lot older than he is. He made no response, no verbal response to anything, just grunted and groaned a lot and slobbered. I thought prob-

ably he would be here for the rest of his life. About a day later someone brought John to the music hour and I saw him sort of stretched
out on a bench like a wet dishcloth. Stevens said to me, "He enjoys
this—he enjoys music very much." I thought to myself, "How utterly
impossible, he isn't even listening to that music." I still thought of
him mostly as a vegetable, but I had the surprised feeling that maybe
there was somebody inside that shell, since Stevens had said he enjoys the music so much. When he tried to kiss me, this was another
indication that there was something human inside that shell.

Ruth felt more comfortable after getting support and encouragement at the staff conference. Her interest in the patient increased as a result of John's response to her talk with him. Ruth
began to see potentialities in the patient that she had not seen
before. She said that curiosity was probably her strongest motivation for trying the suggestions made at the conference. When her
talk with the patient went well, she became increasingly curious
as to how she might help him. She tried to carry on some activities with John whenever she could and also tried to devise ways
of forming a closer relationship with him. Ruth had been talking
with the patient on the ward, had read to him and played simple
games with him, but felt that John was often not fully aware of
what they were doing together. About two weeks after the conference Ruth suggested that she be permitted to take John for a
picnic on the hospital grounds. The head nurse agreed. Ruth
later described her experience with John at the picnic.

> RUTH: The picnic was a great success. There I *really* got a
> further idea of John as a person.
> HEAD NURSE: In what way?
> RUTH: Before we left the building I asked him to please walk
> straight. I didn't really think he would, but when we got outside he
> walked extremely straight. I started to pass the picnic ground and he
> pulled me back. He grabbed the blanket and spread it on the ground
> himself. All this just flabbergasted me. I was utterly amazed but very
> much pleased. He let me know that he was aware of what we were
> doing. This was the most important thing, I think, because until then
> I had partially suspected that he didn't even realize what I was
> doing. And as time went on, after each contact with him I got more
> and more evidence that he was very much aware of what was going
> on.

Although John and Ruth seemed to enjoy each other's company, the relationship was not without difficulties. Ruth found that she sometimes became angry with the patient—that she was especially annoyed with the way he ate. She discussed this with the sociologist.

RUTH: For some reason that I can't discover I become angry with John because of the way he eats. I remember one time he leaned over the coffee table in the living room and grabbed a coffee cup that had a little coffee at the bottom. He started taking it out with his fingers, so I ran over and took the cup away from him.

SOCIOLOGIST: Why were you so angry?

RUTH: I just hated to see him trying to get that last little bit of coffee from somebody else's cup. When I took it from his hands I said, "John, that's not the thing to do, and it makes me very angry to see you do it."

SOCIOLOGIST: You were really being moralistic about it.

RUTH: I certainly gave him a good talking-to. Another time he was eating a peach and dropped it on the floor and then picked it up and began to eat it again. I took it away from him and told him not to eat things off the floor. Another thing that bothers me is his messiness and the way he dawdles over his food.

SOCIOLOGIST: You don't know why you are annoyed?

RUTH: No, I haven't been able to figure it out.

SOCIOLOGIST: I could guess. I think it may have to do with the fact that you are beginning to see that he is capable of more mature behavior and you think, "Why on earth does he do this if he really doesn't have to?"

RUTH: That may be true.

SOCIOLOGIST: But he has to, doesn't he? Because even though he is capable of, say, spreading the blanket as he did on the picnic, he still may have to eat this way. With some things he is able to be more mature, and with other things he is not. Evidently eating and this whole area of food must be terribly important to him. As he gets better this will disappear, but it's going to be a long, hard pull. I can see him straightening up and walking faster and stopping the twitching and grimacing, but I think the last to go may be the hanging onto food and coffee, and the slowness and messiness.

RUTH: Probably you're right about that, but I can't accept his behavior. I'm impatient about it when I'm around him.

SOCIOLOGIST: Well, some things get you down. You might as well recognize them, and the more you know about them the more comfortable you are in dealing with them.

RUTH: I gave myself a long talking-to the other day and decided that come what may I was not going to get angry at John when he dawdles a long time over food and plays with it. But it didn't work. At one point I said, "Come on, John, will you eat your food, please?" With that he picked up a little piece of cake with his fingers and sort of waved it around in the air. I got angry and tried to push him into eating it.

SOCIOLOGIST: Did he eat any faster then?

RUTH: No, he got stubborn. So that's not the best way to handle the situation.

On another occasion Ruth discovered, quite by accident, a way of handling John's eating difficulties. She talked about this with a nurse.

RUTH: I was helping John with his lunch the other day. I wanted to take him to the music hour right afterward because I know he enjoys that. It took him a long time to eat. He played with the food a lot, must have been eating for about an hour and forty-five minutes, and the food got cold, of course. The music was due to start in fifteen minutes, so I said we would have to finish, that's all, and if he couldn't finish it I'd have to take it away. This got him very excited and he started clutching for things. So I thought, well, I hate to do it, but I'll spoon-feed him. And I did. He accepted this very well; he liked it. But I hated to do it. I told him I realized that this was what people do with children and I did not think he was a child, but this was obviously the only way we were going to get the food down him and have him ready in time for the music hour. So he ate very fast with the spoon-feeding. I'm sure anybody could spoon-feed him any time and he would just love it, but I get a guilt feeling. I feel as if I were treating him like a little baby.

Despite her misgivings about spoon-feeding John, Ruth did so occasionally without feeling too uncomfortable because the patient ate better and seemed to enjoy his food more. One day John seemed to want to feed himself, and after that, he continued to eat unassisted. His eating habits improved slightly and Ruth became less annoyed with the way he ate.

Approximately four weeks after the group discussion, personnel commented that John's participation with others had increased and that he was showing definite signs of improvement. Ruth discussed with the sociologist the ways in which the patient participated more actively.

> RUTH: He took part in a picture charade game the other day. He took the pencil and paper and he listened to the name of the song and then tried to draw it, but he was so slow that he couldn't get it done in time. So I suggested that maybe he should try giving the names of the songs to other people. Well, he finally drew a string of pearls and wrote the song title "String of Pearls" alongside.
>
> SOCIOLOGIST: That's very good.
>
> RUTH: So I said, "That's fine." Each time he wrote down the name of the song and then tried to draw it, which I think was excellent. I was amazed.
>
> SOCIOLOGIST: I know he voted for the patient committee. I remember Susan brought a piece of paper to him and he actually chose a name and put a cross in front of it. How did all these changes come about?
>
> RUTH: It seems to me they came about very gradually. He just gradually began to participate in more and more things and his responses became more spontaneous. I was very pleased. I think he has come a long way.
>
> SOCIOLOGIST: In what other ways has he changed?
>
> RUTH: He doesn't go through nearly so much spastic movement as he did previously. He talks a little more.
>
> SOCIOLOGIST: He stands up straight much more often.
>
> RUTH: Walks fast when he wants to, though not all the time.
>
> SOCIOLOGIST: A lot depends on what your focus on the change is— your perspective on it, whether you can see that though these changes seem small, they are important. But he is still very sick.
>
> RUTH: Oh, yes.
>
> SOCIOLOGIST: Sure he's sick, but if you consider the contrast between his behavior now and when you started working with him, you can see quite a few changes. I remember when John was just a sack, a drooling messy sack stretched out in a heap on the floor. When he first used to do this, personnel tried to pick him up, but after a while they just let him lie there. If you consider that and look at him now, there is a significant change, but as you go along each step is very small.

Since communicating with others was a difficult problem for John, Ruth decided on the basis of his activity at the charade game to try to communicate with him through the written word. When John seemed to be trying to talk, Ruth would hand him pencil and paper, saying, "If you can't say it, maybe you can write it." Once she asked him a question verbally and wrote "Yes" and "No" on the pad for him to check. Instead of just checking his answer, John slowly wrote a whole sentence in reply. Because she could communicate a little more easily with the patient, Ruth felt that she understood John better and was able to get a little closer to him.

Ruth's growth in understanding included an appreciation of John's time sense as it differed from her own. She began to understand in a vague way the reason the patient moved so slowly; perhaps the patient did not experience the slowness the same way she did; perhaps the pace at which other people moved was very fast for him. She described one incident that helped her understand his sense of time. Ruth was with John in the ward living room while his sister was visiting him.

RUTH: You know John used to play the piano a great deal. His sister sat down at the piano and began to play, and John got up from his chair and walked over a little way so that he could watch her and then stood there. I got up and took his hand and said, "Do you want to go over to the piano?" He started to move in that direction, but didn't follow through. So I gently led him over to the piano where he stood for a while, and then he bent down alongside his sister, sort of hovering over her.

SOCIOLOGIST: Did he make any move to play?

RUTH: Not at first. Miss Cooper played some more and then she got up and walked away. John stood up but kept hovering over the piano, with a glass in his hand, sipping occasionally. Then he sat down at the piano and put the glass down. He put one hand over the keyboard, and the other he kept waving in the air. By watching his hand I somehow got the idea that he was beckoning to somebody to come, so I went over and stood near him and then sat down with him at the piano. I just sat and waited, and waited, and waited. It seemed like an eternity. But there was something about the way he was looking at that piano that just made me know he was going to play. So I thought, "His concept of time is not the same as mine." Although it seemed to me like an enternity, it was probably a very brief time for John—just a brief moment of decision. I guess I sat there with him for about twenty minutes, in utter silence.

SOCIOLOGIST: Seemed like twenty hours?

RUTH: His sister was getting very nervous at this point and kept making little comments, such as "Would you like to play the piano, John?" I was still sitting there very quietly. Finally, he put one hand over the keyboard again and struck a note. I was so pleased when I heard that note!

SOCIOLOGIST: Just that one note!

RUTH: It was better than any symphony. Sister responded to this note with, "That was very nice, John, why don't you play another note?" I thought to myself, "Why don't you keep still?" John stiffened somewhat when she said that and just sat there, and we both sat another long time. I don't really know how long it was. Finally I said, "If you want to play some more, by all means do, but don't feel that you must play if you don't want to. Maybe you can play tomorrow, and if you don't want to play then, maybe you will feel like playing some other time when your sister comes for a visit." But we sat there a while longer and then I got up because by then I was exhausted.

SOCIOLOGIST: Just by sitting?

RUTH: Yes. So I went over and stood by Miss Cooper. After a long pause, John struck another note on the piano. Sister encouraged him again. She said, "That was very nice, John, why don't you play another one?" John stopped and stiffened again and sat huddled over the piano but didn't play any more.

SOCIOLOGIST: You were really able to identify with John and get his view of the world.

RUTH: I even felt for a few seconds while sitting at the piano for that awfully long time how this must feel to him, that it was just a second, a moment of decision.

SOCIOLOGIST: The twenty minutes appeared to you as you felt they appeared to John, as just one second.

RUTH: I didn't feel that way the whole period because it seemed about three times as long as it really was, but there were seconds during it that I could almost feel the way John felt. I could understand emotionally how he felt.

One of the difficulties Ruth had to face was her concern about getting involved with the patient. When she was forming increasingly close relations with the patient, some of the personnel cautioned her about getting too close to John.

RUTH: It took me a long time to feel that I could get into any sort of real relationship with John. Some of the nurses told me that I should not get involved. I should be more professional and keep my distance.

SOCIOLOGIST: If by involved they mean going out with the patient on dates, that's true and I think it is wise. But if they mean by "involved" that you're not supposed to be human and friendly when you work with mental patients, then you can be sure we are never going to be able to do them any good.

RUTH: I had to reach this decision myself finally. I could see that my relationships with other patients were so extremely superficial that I wasn't feeling like a real person myself. That's not very fair to patients when they need a real person to relate to.

SOCIOLOGIST: You do get something out of your relationship. What are you getting out of it personally?

RUTH: I'm getting a certain amount of prestige out of it. I am able to relate with John, something other people are either not able or not willing to do, and I get a feeling of importance from it which is very satisfying. Also, when I am able to get any sort of response from John, or whenever I hear that he is now doing something he has never done before, this is very satisfying, and I feel I have contributed to this improvement. So that it's undoubtedly a combination of feeling that I am doing a good job and that John is getting something out of it.

SOCIOLOGIST: You also feel good about your relationship with John because you are growing, and because you are able to do all these things for him and with him. You have developed a certain amount of security with John, and you feel pretty good about him. And this is the basic condition, I think, that enables you to help him. Once you feel good about the situation then you can be free enough to follow your feelings without embarrassment, shame, or feeling you are doing something wrong. When you don't feel good about it then you're confused; you don't really know what your feelings are. It is difficult to give intellectual answers to these problems. We can answer them better on the feeling level of what isn't right or appropriate for the situation in terms of what the patient is trying to do and how you feel about it and what your relationship is at the moment. If you hadn't become involved with John, neither of you could have developed to the stage where you are now.

Another problem for Ruth was her discomfort when other personnel were watching her and John engage in some activity. She felt that she had greater freedom to "be herself" when she was not observed by other personnel. When they were around, she became concerned about their attitudes toward her and wondered what they were thinking. The sociologist and head nurse discussed this problem.

HEAD NURSE: Even though Ruth is doing an excellent job with John, she still is insecure about the attitudes of other personnel——especially those who have been here much longer than she has. She's uncomfortable when they watch her with John. She thinks they will be critical.

SOCIOLOGIST: They may just be curious to see what she's doing and also think they might learn something.

HEAD NURSE: It seems that when they watch her she feels more inhibited, as if there were a barrier between her and John.

SOCIOLOGIST: I wonder how we could help her get a sense of inner freedom—help her see that the situation can't be exactly as she would like it to be. Even if some of the others are critical of her, how can we get her to see that she can develop this inner freedom to the point where she feels she can handle the reactions of others without being thrown by them. This is not the same as thinking, "I don't care what other people's reactions are." It is more a feeling of confidence in what she's doing—when if somebody laughs at her she can say to herself, "It's too bad he has to laugh, but I think I'm being helpful, and I can handle the situation in such a way that it won't interfere with my relationship with John." She can't expect to change the environment as much as she can change her own attitude so that she can act with more freedom and spontaneity.

HEAD NURSE: There may be one or two persons on the ward who are so restricted in what they can allow themselves to do with patients that they will be critical if Ruth is a little more spontaneous with John or treats him a little differently. It seems to me she can learn to handle their attitudes without letting them prevent her from using her imagination in dealing with John.

After Ruth had been carrying on this relationship with John for about two months, she had to leave the hospital for personal reasons. She was concerned about the effect of her leaving on John and discussed with the sociologist the best way of telling him that she was going to leave.

RUTH: I want to talk with John and tell him that I'm going to leave soon—not that I want to leave, but that I have to. I really want to stay, but I can't. I'm going to try to make it as clear as possible to him that I'm not rejecting him.

SOCIOLOGIST: He is going to feel the loss; there's no getting away from that. But maybe you can help him reach out for someone else.

Also, you might tell him that you still are fond of him, and that you're not going to change your feelings toward him just because you are leaving.

A few days after Ruth had told John about her leaving she talked with the sociologist again.

RUTH: When I told John I was leaving he seemed to be hurt, but I was able to help him make some contact with the new aide, Phyllis. Just today we were playing a game and Phyllis came out and played with us, and John grabbed hold of Phyllis, took her back with him, and just left me. I really felt rejected. I didn't think I should feel rejected, you know, but I knew that deep down inside I did.

SOCIOLOGIST: There is no sense in deceiving yourself. If you feel that way, you just do. I think, however, part of your feeling may be related to the fact that you are leaving. It's been a pretty good experience for you and you are ending it now.

RUTH: I don't want it to end.

SOCIOLOGIST: Maybe you can get used to the idea that whatever you contributed to John is already part of him. So whatever he does with anybody else, the part of him that is your contribution is *doing* it. He's building on this in the same way a child builds on what his mother gives him, so that he can reach out and develop relationships with other people. I think that's true, and it takes the edge off the feeling that all your contribution is ended. You may feel, too, that you're not going to learn any more—that your learning process has ended, at least about John's behavior.

RUTH: That's true.

SOCIOLOGIST: But again, what you have gained from him is not lost, and what he has given you—your own growth and development and your ability to see and understand people—is not lost. Whatever you build on in that direction will be, at least in part, contributed to by what John did for you. I wonder if you could possibly give this new aide some of the ideas and knowledge you have accumulated in such a way that she can accept them.

RUTH: I have already talked to Phyllis a little, and she doesn't seem very enthusiastic about doing much with John. She wanted to know how she could get out of the situation. She said John was getting too fond of her. I advised her to discuss it at the ward staff conference and wait to see if she really wants to get out of it.

SOCIOLOGIST: I certainly wouldn't push her to develop a closer relationship with John. But you might describe what happened to you—that you had your doubts and how your attitudes changed.

RUTH: I don't think she wants to reject him. I have a feeling that she does want to deal with him in the most effective way she can in the situation, but I think she is just not willing to face it yet.

SOCIOLOGIST: Maybe it will take a little time. It's interesting to ask: How did your attitude change? If you go over your experience here, you will see a gradual change in your feelings and in your attitudes about your relationship with John, and a change in what you were able to feel and see about him and in what you were able to be with him. Some of this happens outside of your deliberate intentions to do it. There is a gradual evolution of the changed attitude. You can't put your finger on any particular thing and say, "This did it," but you can pick out particular factors that are part of the whole picture—your own motivation and curiosity, your getting some support at the staff conference, getting the feeling as you went along that there is something worthwhile here that you could get and that you could give. One crucial thing, I think, was the staff conference. Would you agree with that?

RUTH: I think I would go along with that.

SOCIOLOGIST: I think that permitted everything else to develop. I think that if you had not been given some help in that conference, you probably would have been pretty unhappy and would have been quite anxious with John.

RUTH: I probably would have eventually pulled out of it. This feeling of support was very necessary.

SOCIOLOGIST: So you got it from the group, and then you were able to develop yourself. This question of how attitudes change is a very central problem, I think, because, after all, these attitudes are the foundations for our ways of relating to people. If you can change them, you can change your relationships. If we can get some idea of what was important in your experience with John, it may throw a little more light on our understanding of how attitudes become changed and what we can do to help change them in a useful direction.

The preceding example illustrates a number of interpersonal aspects of the nurse-patient relationship that we will discuss in subsequent chapters. We note here that nursing personnel placed great importance on and devoted an entire conference to trying to *understand the patient*: that is, they tried to determine what needs the patient was seeking to have fulfilled when he clung to the aide and attempted to have physical contact with her. As the aide began to see the patient as more of a human being, she

became more friendly toward him; she developed greater understanding of him and increased her awareness of what it means to
be a patient.

Throughout the relationship the aide was trying to *communicate
with the patient*. This was difficult, since the patient rarely used
words. But the aide at one point discovered that they could
exchange a little more through written communication. Despite
this, there was still a great deal of difficulty in carrying on meaningful exchange, especially in any continuous way.

Initially the patient's physical approaches to her made the aide
uncomfortable and *anxious in relating to the patient*. She tried to
overcome her anxiety by *setting limits* on the patient's behavior
(trying to prevent him from touching her). Her verbal prohibitions did not succeed. Only when she changed her feelings and
her approach to the patient did he give up this behavior, and
only then did her anxiety decrease markedly.

Increasing familiarity with the patient and continuing relations with him enabled the aide to develop greater *sensitivity to the
patient*. This was strikingly demonstrated when the patient tried
to play the piano. At that time the aide was able to identify with
the patient and gain an appreciation of his internal struggle in
trying to play; she also got some idea of the patient's conception
of time and how it seemed to differ from her own. In addition,
increasing familiarity meant increasing *respect for the patient*. The
aide began to see how the patient might change and develop
more mature behavior. As the patient did change, the aide began
to wonder if this meant he was improving. She began to look for
ways to *identify patient improvement* and to ask herself how the
significance of the improvement could be evaluated.

Although the relationship between the aide and the patient
was, in general, a good one, it was not without difficulties for the
aide. One of these difficulties was her annoyance and anger with
the patient because of his eating habits. The aide's *conventional
attitudes and expectations* interfered with her being helpful to the
patient during mealtime. When she was able to handle this
problem more successfully and began to spoon-feed the patient,
the aide became concerned about whether she was *treating the*

patient as a child. She wondered if she were being disrespectful to the patient and helping to keep him in a childlike state. She discovered that with her willingness to help him in this way the patient could go on to more mature behavior. She faced another problem when she was cautioned by other personnel *not to get involved with the patient.* They implied that if she were warm and friendly toward the patient she was in some way being unprofessional, or might get in "too deep" and not know how to get out. She discovered that she could be warm and friendly with the patient, and because of this friendliness she was able to perform more effectively as an aide.

Understanding the Patient

IT is difficult to generalize about mental patients because they
vary so much in their dynamics and in the manifestations of
their illness. It is also difficult to make definitive and conclusive
statements about the origin, functioning, and cure of *functional
mental illness*. Our understanding of the causes of mental illness is
incomplete; there are many uncertainties and obscurities in our
knowledge of the way it operates; we still have much to learn
about treating and curing the mentally ill. Nevertheless, the
recognition and appreciation by the nurse of what we do know
about mental patients could increase her understanding of individual patients. However, the conceptions we present are just a
small part of the knowledge that has been gathered about mental
patients, and it is not our intent that they be used by the nurse
as a substitute for learning about patients through her relations
with them. Only through such experience can she test the validity
or applicability of our conceptions. In continuing exchange with
patients she can acquire understanding of them, test the adequacy
of her understanding, grow in her understanding, and put her
understanding into operation for the welfare of the patient and
for greater satisfaction for herself.

A CONCEPTION OF MENTAL ILLNESS

What do we mean when we say a person is mentally ill? We
mean that he is so uncomfortable and so severely disturbed in his
relations with other people that he has to be segregated and
placed in a special environment in order to protect both him and
them. Our view is that mental illness is not a disease that a patient "has" in the same way that he has a virus infection or an

organic lesion; rather, mental illness is the way the patient thinks, believes, and feels about other people and the way he acts with them. His difficulties in living are so severe and his anxiety so great that he is incapacitated or ineffective in his relations with others. His behavior may be so deviant as to be conspicuous, troublesome, puzzling, and painful for both the patient and others, or he may be so withdrawn that others become worried about him or find it difficult to relate to him in a satisfying way. In effect, confusion, lack of understandable communication, assaultiveness, hallucinations, delusions, panic, or withdrawn behavior—*the patient's distinctive and characteristic ways of participating with others—are his mental illness.* In other words, the patient's mental illness is his pattern of participation in interpersonal relations—his typical and regular ways of relating to others. However, these "sick" ways of dealing with others are only a part, although an outstanding part, of the patient's personality. Another very important part, not so easily seen but nevertheless there, is the patient's "drive toward health." Each patient has a tendency—a striving—to "get better." This tendency is present in all patients, and in those who remain ill it awaits the conditions, situations, and interpersonal relations that will nourish it, develop and mobilize it, and bring it to the fore. In working with the patient in a therapeutic direction the nurse builds upon and facilitates the growth of this tendency toward health.

A common conception in our society is that the mentally ill person is a different order of being ("something less than human") from the rest of us. Psychiatrists[1] have shown that the mentally ill person is not so completely different from the non-psychotic person. They have also indicated that "we are all more simply human than otherwise." The psychotic person uses the same kinds of mental processes that we use, but in a somewhat different way, with his own unique emphasis or twist. He may have an exaggerated reaction to a situation or a feeling about it

---

[1] We have relied for our point of view primarily on the writings and teachings of Dr. Harry Stack Sullivan and Dr. Frieda Fromm-Reichmann. See, for example, Sullivan, Harry Stack, *The Interpersonal Theory of Psychiatry*, edited by Helen S. Perry and Mary L. Gawel, W. W. Norton and Co., New York, 1953; and Fromm-Reichmann, Frieda, *Principles of Intensive Psychotherapy*, University of Chicago Press, Chicago, 1950.

that is unwarranted, or he may distort reality to fit his own ideas and preconceptions. But the difference between his mental operations and behavior and those of the nonpsychotic person is primarily one in degree and not in kind. The line between the two may not be sharp or clear, and the distinction is more a quantitative than a qualitative one. In addition, when a person is mentally ill he is not completely or totally psychotic, nor is he "sick" all of the time. Only select aspects of him are sick, and he acts in a psychotic way only at certain times. However, he participates with sick behavior sufficiently frequently, in a variety of situations, to be labeled "psychotic."

Although we cannot measure degree of illness accurately, we view people as being mentally healthy in varying degrees; no one is completely "sick," nor is anyone completely healthy. Each of us performs in ways that can be considered more or less mentally healthy. Similarly, variations in degree of mental health can be seen in the same person over a period of time. Thus, the patient can be seen to be performing more adequately and appropriately in some situations than he does in others.

There are other aspects of our point of view that are in sharp contrast to many common conceptions of the mental patient. *The mentally ill person is not hopeless*, even if he has been hospitalized for many years. He has remarkable capacities and potentialities for change. We can relate and communicate with him, and we can be realistically hopeful for his improvement if we have the ingenuity and patience to discover the most effective ways of bringing change about. *The mentally ill person is not "bad,"* and it is inappropriate to judge him according to moral standards. The patient cannot "help" what he is doing in many situations, and a moral or judgmental attitude toward behavior he cannot "control" is only likely to reinforce it. *The mentally ill person is not "deliberately" acting the way he does.* He is desperately trying to handle and to minimize his severe distress, and his characteristic behavior is one way he has of doing this. A view that is much more realistic and useful is that the patient is a sick person who needs to be helped to help himself, and that this can only come about in a gradual way, with difficulty and backsliding before improvement is solidified. In this process the patient needs consistent respect and acceptance. Finally, we need neither overestimate nor underestimate the importance of any one experience for the patient. *He is neither so delicate that one experience will devastate him nor is he so insensitive that he will be unaffected by any one experience.* The patient has resilience and a good capacity for survival, but at the same time he can be deeply affected and disturbed by what others do with him. He especially may be affected by relations with nursing personnel that continue over a long period of time.

Implicit in our point of view is the idea that the patient has become mentally ill as a result of the kinds of experiences he has had. *It follows from this that his illness can be influenced, interrupted, and altered by what other people do to and with him.* For the nurse in the mental hospital, this means that what she and her colleagues do with patients, the kinds of relations they carry on with them, can be of great significance in helping the patient to mental health. We can see why nurse-patient relations are of great importance if we remember that nurses are in continuous, close, and emotionally important relations with patients and, for the most part, constitute the persistent, real, and immediate personal environment for them. If the nurse is to make optimum use of the opportunity afforded her to change the patient's mental illness and facilitate his mental health, she must develop and act on greater understanding of the patient, herself, and the kinds of interpersonal relations they maintain with each other.

What It Means to Be a Patient

Although it is difficult to convey in words what it means to be a mental patient, we will attempt to do this, first by trying to describe his thoughts and feelings, then by looking at the meaning of mental illness in our society, and finally by seeing what it means to be in a mental hospital. All that we describe here is not necessarily part of the experience of every patient, but many patients have had a great number of these experiences.

The inner life of the patient is chaotic. He is not clear what his illness *is* nor what he must do to *get better*. He is confused about the boundaries between himself and other people—where he begins and ends and where other people begin and end. He is vague and confused about what he is, what he ought to be and what he could be. He feels that he is made up of separate parts that do not fit together. He is not sure what comes out of him (that is, what is a product of his own efforts) and what comes to him from the outside. The patient is uncertain about the effects of his actions or whether they have any effect at all. He is quite fearful of his surroundings, but most of all he is afraid and distrustful of himself. Will he do something dangerous to himself or to others? Is he something less than human because he is mentally ill? Will he be able to control his behavior, or will "it" control him and force him to do horrible things? He is filled with anxiety and loneliness. He feels, "Does anyone really care? Who in the wide world has felt such unrelieved misery, such utter abandonment, loneliness, desperation, and isolation from the rest of mankind?" The anxiety he experiences can be paralyzing, terrifying, or just severe enough to make him feel exceedingly uncomfortable with other people, but it is almost always a constant companion. He is also distrustful and suspicious of the intentions of others toward him— suspicious that they might want to injure him. The patient feels he is a defeated person, a failure in living with others, incapable of running his own life or assuming responsibility. With this defeat come feelings of unworthiness, hopelessness, helplessness, and resentment and hatred toward others whom he believes responsible for his condition or who are "well" while he is "sick." He feels guilty about his strong negative feelings and fears he will be punished for them.

The patient has strong feelings of insecurity and inferiority. He is afraid of being ignored, rejected, or slighted, and is easily hurt when he is so treated. Yet he may feel embarrassed when he is singled out in a way that makes him conspicuous. He fears that others may be contemptuous of him, and he might try to be contemptuous first or he might give the impression that he is unaffected by the attitudes of others toward him. The patient is frequently confused and severely distorts his environment. He may see objects differently from the way we see them—as smaller

or larger than they are, as possessing human powers, as controlling or threatening him. He may mix up time, places, and persons.
Sometimes he feels that a great wall or distance separates him
from everyone else, and he may feel frozen in the presence of
others. People may appear to move around without cause, reason,
or purpose, as he feels he does. Hanging over him is a sense of
being doomed to continue in a state of misery, discontent, and
dread.

Persons outside of mental hospitals have experienced many of
these feelings at one time or another. The mental patient experiences them more often and more intensely, with less hope of
overcoming them and with less confidence that he will be able
to handle them adequately. However, the patient also experiences
cooperative, tender, kindly, and other satisfying feelings. These
occur less frequently, are more fleeting and more difficult to
evoke. An important aspect of the mentally ill person is the
internal conflict he experiences in the area of warm, tender,
loving human relations. On the one hand, the patient has an
intense and desperate need for acceptance, support, and understanding—a great need to be cared about in a genuine way and
to share tenderness and affection with another. He also despairs
that this will ever happen, since it has happened so rarely in the
past. On the other hand, the patient sometimes openly manifests
rejection of and hatred toward others, driving away the person
who attempts to provide some of this affection. The patient wants
to be close to another, but at the same time he may attack the
person with whom he is forming a close relationship. If the nurse
recognizes that the patient is afraid of closeness to another person,
she may be able to accept these attacks when they occur. Such
recognition might help her see that he runs away because he is
afraid that he might be disappointed and hurt in the relationship.
The tendency to avoid what he wants and to engage in self-
defeating behavior—to ensure that he will not get what he wants
so very much—is a characteristic pattern. Too often the nurse
recognizes only the rejecting overt behavior and finds it difficult
to see the desperate need and desire on the part of the patient
for close and satisfying exchange.

One might justifiably ask: How do we know this need and desire are really there when we see so much of the opposite? The answer to this question is twofold. First, we assume that all persons in order to survive must have had some tenderness and love in the course of being brought up.[1] These experiences constitute the healthy aspect of the personality. Because these tender experiences have been interrupted, infrequent, and insufficient, the patient seeks them again and again. He cannot go about his quest in a simple and direct manner because the search is attended with much anxiety and fear of failure.

Second, nurses have heard about and observed situations in which the patient has, under appropriate circumstances and with particular persons, openly revealed his tender side and has pointedly said that his need for loving and tender relations with others is one of his most desperate needs. Thus, in caring for the mentally ill it is important that the nurse not be turned away by the patient's rejecting behavior. Behind it are potentialities for warm, responsive behavior that can be reached by the nurse if she recognizes and seeks to understand these hidden aspects of the patient. If she persists in offering him a warm, respectful relationship, he may come to trust her and have less need to attack her or withdraw from close relations. The nurse may discover that she can derive much gratification from seeing their relationship grow.

A common and widespread attitude in our society is that the mentally ill person is dangerous to himself or others and, therefore, should be locked up. The mental patient rejects many of our society's standards and conventions, and we, in turn, reject him because he does not abide by them. In addition, we attach a stigma to being mentally ill. We feel that psychosis is something shameful, and, therefore, families often try to keep the patient's illness a secret. The idea of associating with "crazy people" makes us uncomfortable, and we tend to avoid them. There is a feeling of dread about mental illness or a mental hospital, but at the same time we feel a certain fascination and curiosity about the

---

[1] For evidence supporting this assumption, see Ribble, Margaret, *The Rights of Infants*, Columbia University Press, New York, 1943; and Spitz, René A., "Hospitalism," *The Psychoanalytic Study of the Child*, International Universities Press, New York, vol. 1, 1945, pp. 53–74.

mentally ill. Not only do people, in general, feel that a psychosis is a disgraceful illness and that the mentally ill are inferior people who are not to be trusted, but patients have these attitudes toward themselves and each other. For patients, too, have adopted our cultural attitudes toward mental illness.

There are other attitudes toward the mentally ill in our society. There is humanitarian concern and interest in ameliorating their lot and in helping them to better health. Understanding of the conditions that bring mental illness about is developing and we are applying psychiatric and social science knowledge in the treatment of the mentally ill, though as yet society does not provide sufficient funds to make mental hospitals the kinds of therapeutic institutions they can be.

Our attitudes toward the mentally ill person are a mixture of fear and desire to punish him, guilt about him, protection of him, pity and sympathy for him, desire to understand him, and concern about alleviating his condition. With this ambivalence we erect mental hospitals, sometimes forgetting what the hospital means to the patient. We may overlook the fact that we deprive the mental patient of freedom of movement and other freedoms that we take for granted ourselves. We segregate him with others who appear to be like himself, but who might be frightening to him. We take away his responsibility for himself and for the conduct of his own life: he is told when to come and go, when to eat, when to go to sleep, when to get out of bed, and so on. Because he has not been able to direct his life in a useful, productive, and socially acceptable way outside the hospital, we assume that he cannot make any decisions that will be for his benefit inside the hospital. *We do not test this assumption often enough.* Instead, the mental hospital staff takes responsibility for him, regulates and directs his life. On the one hand, some routine, order, and regularity might be of value to a mental patient who has led a disorganized life. Protecting the patient and organizing his surroundings may make him feel more secure. On the other hand, at times he may be made to feel like a prisoner or a child.

It must be remembered that the patient's life is unavoidably regulated by strangers and that he is forced to live among them despite his wishes. In a mental institution the patient has little, if any, privacy. Mental hospitals too often deal with patients in an impersonal way, looking upon them as part of a mass rather than as unique individuals who have separate identities and whose individuality should be respected. Thus, it seems that societal attitudes and the organization of mental hospitals present many difficulties for the mental patient which may only add to his burden. Of course, the mental hospital is also helpful to the mental patient. It is hard to tell how great a contribution the hospital makes toward the patient's improvement, or whether in some cases a patient improves despite the hospital rather than because of it. The nurse's function is to maximize her helpfulness to the patient within the limits set by the hospital and to suggest changes in these limits where therapeutic benefit might result for the patient.

The Patient's Needs

What does a patient need from the nurse, and how can she understand and meet his needs? We have discussed patient needs in a general way in previous chapters. Here we will bring together some of the ideas mentioned before and try to present a simple yet meaningful explanation of the patient's needs, recognizing that the needs of patients can be looked at in many different ways and that we are omitting many complexities.

In order to survive biologically and maintain his physical well-being the patient needs food, water, sleep, clothing, shelter, and so on; he needs to be protected against physical injury and illness and given proper medical care when these occur.

Second, at any particular time a patient may have specific needs, such as, for a cigarette, an item of clothing, a game, a walk, or a conversation with another person. These needs are concrete and might be easily understood if the patient could express himself. Many patients have difficulty in indicating their needs and hope that the nurse will discover what they are. The importance of understanding the patient's specific needs and fulfilling them if possible lies not only in the immediate gratification the patient gets, but also in the fact that in understanding and fulfilling his needs the nurse indicates that she cares about meeting them. Supplying a simple object that the patient needs might be of considerable significance to the patient who does not think he deserves it, who has been frequently frustrated, and who is afraid to hope that he can have his needs understood and fulfilled.

Third, the patient needs to feel worthwhile and appreciated. This means he needs tenderness and affection. He needs to be liked, approved of, accepted, respected, attended to, and made to feel that he counts and that someone cares about him. Patients notably have derogatory and contemptuous attitudes toward themselves and do not believe they are important enough really to matter to anyone. A patient may desperately want the nurse to contradict the low opinion he has of himself by appreciating him and making him feel that she considers him worthwhile.

Fourth, the patient needs to participate with others and form a relationship with them. Although some patients give the impression of preferring their isolation, many if not all patients have an intense need to decrease their loneliness and be related to another person in a satisfying way. In fulfilling his need for intimacy and companionship in a way that is acceptable to the patient, the nurse must take into account the patient's fears in relating with another and his disbelief that he can get some gratification from it. Despite the fact that he needs participation with another, a patient may prefer loneliness to taking the chance that his need for the nurse's companionship will be ignored, rebuffed, overlooked, contemptuously denied, or that the relationship will turn out to be painful.

Fifth, the patient needs to communicate with another person. He needs to talk with someone, to be understood and to understand the other, to exchange ideas, and to share thoughts and feelings.

Finally, the patient needs to be free from overwhelming anxiety. He needs to feel a measure of inner security and equilibrium. He needs to have his anxiety sufficiently decreased so that he is not in a constant state of distress.

It is obvious that the needs we have listed are overlapping—that ignoring or fulfilling one means that another is ignored or fulfilled. For example, when the patient gets a cigarette from the nurse he may also feel worthwhile because he has been attended to and has, in addition, been able to have a brief exchange with the nurse. When the nurse talks with the patient, when she bathes him or gives him medication, she may be giving him support and approval at the same time. When the nurse feeds the patient or plays a game with him, she may make him feel worthwhile, increase his comfort, and reduce his anxiety. Of course, it does not necessarily follow that various needs are fulfilled simultaneously. The opposite may be true: one need may be met when another is not. For example, if the nurse feels disgusted and rejecting of the patient while she is feeding him, the patient is receiving food but he may not feel worthwhile in this process.

The needs we have been describing are human needs that all of us have. In general, the patient has suffered much greater frustration of his needs than we have. His mental illness is due, at least in part, to this lack of fulfillment. In addition, because of this deprivation in his past the patient has considerable anxiety concerning his needs. In the past, others have misunderstood, ignored, or deliberately not fulfilled his needs. He, therefore, may be reluctant to make an effort to get them fulfilled. He is also afraid to let himself feel dependent on the nurse because he anticipates that he may be rebuffed again. Even though he may experience his needs intensely and his wish for their gratification may be great, he may be unable to admit this to himself or to the nurse. The anxiety aroused by the possibility of severe disappointment makes denial of his needs preferable to "taking a chance" on being unfulfilled. Sometimes when he feels a need intensely he may try desperately to get the nurse to help him, but he may do it in such a way that he antagonizes the nurse or in some way defeats himself and ensures his not receiving what he needs from her. The patient may have to continue to defeat the nurse for a time and prevent her from meeting his needs even though this means he is defeating himself. The patient may seek immediate gratification of his needs, may be impatient with any delay, may have difficulty in sustaining any kind of frustration, and even when his needs are met may have difficulty in deriving gratification from their fulfillment.

The patient may have other problems in getting his needs fulfilled. He may be inexperienced, awkward, and ineffective in making his needs known. He may ask for something in a way that is unacceptable to the nurse or communicate his needs in unconventional and unexpected ways. Or he may have difficulty in communicating his needs in a simple, clear, direct, and understandable way; instead, he may obscure what he needs by asking for something else, or he may express his needs in a vague, confused manner. Sometimes he does not or cannot verbalize his needs at all.

The patient may also be in conflict about his needs. On the one hand, he may intensely want the gratification of a need and be motivated to do something about it. On the other hand, he is afraid to hope for or expect anything from the nurse; he is afraid to trust her or have faith in her. He feels he is not worthy enough to have his needs met and thus shies away from making any effort on his own behalf. Because he is uncertain that anyone is "really interested" in him, he may "feel" his way and be very hesitant in indicating his needs to the nurse. He may hint vaguely about what he wants, to see if the nurse "catches on." He may wait for reassurance that it is "all right" to ask to have his needs fulfilled. Some such inner conflict may account for a situation in which a patient vacillates between accepting and rejecting the nurse's attempt to fulfill his need. Thus, he may reject or attack the very person he is hoping desperately will meet his need.

In short, in attempting to fulfill their needs, patients will reveal their inner conflicts, their distortions, their suspicions, their distrust, and their anxiety. Despite the patient's doubts, despite past disappointments and deprivations, the patient struggles to make his needs manifest. He works out a pattern of communication (verbal and nonverbal), which is his way of drawing attention to his needs. This pattern may not be the most effective one, but the nurse must discover and understand it in order to work out appropriate ways of meeting his needs.

The nurse's function is to understand the patient's needs, to understand his feelings about them, and to try to fulfill them in an appropriate way. How might the nurse do this? If she is to meet the patient's needs effectively, she must develop *sensitivity to him and his needs.* By trying to put herself in the patient's place imaginatively and emotionally, she might be able to identify a particular need at a particular time, to determine which need is paramount at the moment, and to gain some appreciation of the meaning of the patient's needs to him. She might be able to develop her sensitivity by "leaving herself open" to the patient, by paying close attention to her own feelings as she relates to the patient, and by noticing the vague cues she gets from him. Increasing familiarity with the patient will help her discover the patient's ways of expressing his needs and acceptable ways of meeting them.

An earnest desire to meet his needs whenever this is possible and consistent with the patient's welfare might be helpful to the patient. It may be necessary for the nurse to prove over and over again that she is interested in the patient and in providing for his needs before he will come to trust her. The patient may experience the nurse's irritation, annoyance, stereotyped or routine responses to his needs, or a contemptuous or condescending manner as indications of lack of interest in meeting his needs.

When the nurse is trying to decide what the patient needs from her, one course to follow is to accept at face value whatever request the patient makes and then attempt to discover if the patient wants or needs more or something other than what he has indicated.

Even though the nurse's ultimate goal is to have the patient assume more responsibility for meeting his own needs and rely less on others, she may have to accept the patient's extreme dependence on her for a time. Only gradually will he be able to give up this extreme dependence. If the nurse can gratify the patient's needs in ways that are appropriate and acceptable to him at the time, she may help him feel that life is more worthwhile and that there is some possibility for satisfactions in living. In this way she may mobilize his "tendency toward health" and may contribute to his assuming full responsibility for the conduct of his own life.

« 13 »

Communicating with the Patient

ONE of the functions of psychiatric nursing is to facilitate the patient's communication, that is, to help the patient engage in an understandable exchange with the nurse. Since the patient's mental illness is, in part, a defect in communication, it can be expected that the nurse will have difficulty understanding the patient's communication; he, in turn, will have difficulty understanding the nurse and making himself understood.

Before we discuss some of the problems involved in nurse-patient communication, we should make it clear that we are not referring only to verbal communication. From one point of view, the patient is *telling the nurse something by everything he says and does;* and the same might be said about the nurse's behavior with the patient. Gestures, stance, a glance, as well as actual words, convey meaning. Thus, when two persons are in contact, communication is continuous. The problem becomes one of interpreting and understanding gestures and words.

Even the slightest understanding between the nurse and patient and even a small amount of meaningful exchange may be important for the patient. It may help him feel that he is not "completely crazy," since he can understand another person and can make himself understood, at least some of the time. In addition, the experience of being understood and understanding another, even if it is about the simplest matters, may be of great importance to a patient who does not take the world and its meanings for granted as we do. That is, as we have pointed out, time, places, and objects may be seen by the patient in ways that are quite different from those in which we see them. When the patient and nurse view the same situation alike, there is a sharing

231

of experience which patients have all too infrequently. Each experience of successful communicative exchange may implant in the patient an expectation that similar experiences may possibly occur again; and this expectation lays the foundation for their recurrence. With the accumulation of partially successful communicative exchanges, more conventional and understandable communication by the patient gradually may emerge, and the patient's feeling that he is so different from everyone else or so "crazy" that he will never be understood may be decreased.

LISTENING TO AND FOCUSING UPON THE PATIENT

On first thought, the nurse may believe that *listening to a patient and becoming actively aware of him* requires no special effort. She may believe that she does this naturally, but we have found that this is not necessarily so. There are many things that interfere with the nurse's becoming an effective listener. It might be helpful to the nurse for us to mention at this point some of the ways she can develop her ability to listen to and focus on the patient.

The nurse's training ordinarily does not teach her how to listen attentively to the patient's words; it teaches her instead how to "do things" for patients and gives her a conception of nursing as a "doing" profession. In listening, the nurse holds in abeyance the necessity for actively doing something and accepts the idea that listening itself is "doing something" for the patient.

There are other reasons why a nurse finds it difficult to listen to a patient while he is talking. The way the patient talks may be a problem for her. The patient may be vague in his talk and the nurse may be unable to follow him; not understanding what he has said, she dismisses it as "nonsense." He may speak so rapidly that it is difficult to attend to his stream of words. The nurse becomes uncomfortable because of the patient's manner or style of delivery. The patient may be so insistent upon the nurse's listening to him that the nurse gets impatient, annoyed, or angry, and is unable to listen. He may talk so much that he does not give the nurse a chance to respond and her attention wanders. His talk may be repetitious and uninteresting, and the nurse gets bored. The patient may make her feel stupid because she is unable to understand what he says, and she becomes resentful. The nurse senses that the feelings underlying the patient's talk are hostile and rejects the patient by not listening to him. The patient's talk may arouse anxiety in her, and she becomes preoccupied with her own feelings and loses sight of what the patient is saying. She feels unable to listen to "crazy talk" because she has the preconception that she will not understand the patient and thinks it is useless to listen to him.

Other patients are hesitant and slow in their speech. They talk so slowly that it is easy for the nurse to become impatient and not wait and listen. It might be important to accept the patient's talk at its slow pace, to reply in the same pace, and to refrain from urging him to talk faster. Some patients are deeply preoccupied with their own talk and thoughts and have considerable difficulty hearing what the nurse is saying. Because these patients are difficult to reach, the nurse may have to repeat a statement slowly and simply a number of times before the patient absorbs its meaning.

A patient's words may have the usually accepted meaning, and, in addition, have connotations that are not readily apparent. For example, the patient may say, "I'm cold and need a hot water bottle," and may mean both that he is cold and that the nurse is too impersonal and distant with him. Sometimes the nurse may think she understands the meaning "behind his words" but may be uncertain about the interpretation in regard to herself. When the nurse finds it difficult to understand the patient, she need not become discouraged even if her confusion and lack of understanding continue. *Focusing upon the patient is in itself a significant response to him.* It may be that the patient is trying to relate to the nurse and that her *listening to him and trying to understand him* is enough to make him feel worthwhile. His frustration at being unable to make himself understood and the nurse's disappointment in not understanding may be less important than the fact of their being together and trying to work out a communicative exchange.

If a patient does not talk, the nurse may have even greater difficulty in focusing on him; that is, she may find it difficult to stay with him in silence and to attend to his nonverbal communication. Ordinarily, the nurse is not used to this kind of activity, and she may be made uncomfortable by it. She tends to experience silence as "hanging heavily" around her and may feel she is wasting her time just sitting quietly when she might be "doing something" useful with another patient. The reasons the nurse finds a patient's silence difficult may be quite diverse. Perhaps she cannot understand why he is mute; she may think he is "deliberately not talking." She may feel inadequate because she thinks "she ought to be able to get the patient to talk" and feels she is a failure if she cannot.

Listening to the patient is essential to creating a situation in which the patient feels free to express himself in whatever form he can at the moment. Giving him an opportunity to express himself and listening attentively may enable the nurse to build a bridge to the patient's world. A nurse who is able to listen carefully may discover that listening is an important step toward a more understandable exchange. Once the nurse has accepted the value of listening patiently, once she gives the patient an opportunity to be heard and to express himself, she may find that she understands more of his communication and that he, in turn, understands her better. With this bridge, the nurse may be able to develop a relatively stable communicative relationship in which the patient and she understand each other in areas that are significant to both. In addition, if the patient feels free to talk about his difficulties, he may not have to act them out; talking about his feelings and thoughts may make it unnecessary for him to engage in behavior that will be harmful to himself or others.

What is the process of attending to the patient whether he talks or not? Much is communicated by the patient without words. When the nurse is focusing on the patient, she is trying to "hear" his nonverbal communication; empathically and intuitively, she is trying to become aware of the patient's feelings and meanings, receiving the information his body movements convey to her and recognizing the unconscious adjustment they are making to each other.

The nurse can increase the extent to which she is focusing on the patient if she is attentive to and deliberately seeks out the non-verbal signs of what the patient is thinking, feeling, and telling her. Ordinarily, these signs will not be obvious. The nurse will have to look for them, but she can learn how to be sensitive to the subtle cues the patient gives her about his inner world.

With the mute patient the nurse can focus her attention exclusively on his nonverbal behavior, which means that she observes carefully, closely, and freely the cues he transmits. When she does this, she might discover that instead of receiving no communication from the patient, she is receiving a great deal. Instead of "time being wasted" during these silent periods, the nurse may find she is putting her time to excellent use when she tries to understand what the patient is conveying by his relaxed or tense muscle tone, the pale or flushed color of his skin, the way he tilts his body, the extent to which his eyes are open, the speed of his movements, the way he looks at her, the position of his feet and arms, the way he shifts and supports his body. These indicators and many others tell the nurse something about the patient, if she can observe and accept them as beginning stages in understanding him. Observing these indicators consists in noticing and thinking about them in order to discover what they mean and how they are related to what is occurring between the patient and nurse at a particular time. The nurse can also develop sensitivity to the nonverbal cues of patients who talk. With these patients the nurse also has to take into account the significance of their words, how they are spoken (inflection, volume, continuity), and how they affect her as a listener. Thus, she listens both to the words and to what is communicated by means other than words.

Listening to and focusing on a patient means that the nurse is an observer who is able to concentrate on what is happening to and within the patient, to and within herself, and between her and the patient. This kind of concentration involves attentive alertness. It means that the nurse keeps herself open and free to hear the patient, that she uses all her senses to take in what is being conveyed, that she is prepared to receive what the patient is transmitting, that she is also listening to the thoughts and feelings aroused in her and evaluating them for the light they might shed on the patient's communication, and that she tries to imagine herself in the patient's place in order to hear him better. If the nurse listens in this alert and responsive way, the chances are increased that the patient will feel that she recognizes and appreciates his desire to be heard. This may encourage him to try to make himself heard.

This process of observation involves an attitude of acceptance and receptivity to the patient's communication. It means that the nurse waits for the patient's communication, that she "goes along with" or follows his communicative leads, and that she takes the cue from the patient instead of directing the communicative situation. This acceptance is in contrast to the impatience a nurse might show when she wants the patient to stop talking so she can talk, or when she wants to leave the patient or proceed with a task she has set for herself. If the nurse insists upon having the communication go in the direction of her interest, she may evoke resistance or negativism. The patient's resistance will then only make it harder for the nurse to listen. Acceptance means she does not have to push him to talk, is under no compulsion to "have a conversation," and can listen in silence. By being free to listen she tries to provide a situation that will encourage the patient to communicate and tries to afford him the opportunity to do so. By her approach the nurse indicates to the patient that she understands that he has to communicate in his own way and in his own good time, and that she can accept this kind of exchange and thereby accept the patient.

If listening to a patient is to be effective, the nurse must sustain her efforts. Interruptions and the nurse's difficulties in concentrating on the patient are quickly noticed by him, with the result that he may be reluctant to continue the exchange. Continued listening does not mean that the nurse necessarily understands what is being communicated. She may be "in the dark" about much of it, but the fact that she is listening may help the patient feel that he is respected. If the nurse's attitude and actions indicate that she feels it is important for the patient to be listened to, he may get some feeling of being attended to and being thought worthwhile. It may be well to remember that there are times when the patient attempts some communication with the nurse, not primarily because he wants to give the nurse a specific message but because he wants some attention, some companionship, or wants to "sound off" to someone.

Listening to a patient is not easy. Patients may make it difficult for the nurse to listen when they talk in an apparently meaningless way, when they are persistently silent, or when they talk rapidly and uninterruptedly. Listening is not easy because it requires time, which the nurse may not have or may not think she has; patience, which is difficult to have when she is anxious or harassed; and interest, which is hard to develop and maintain when her feelings get in her way. But listening, even if only for a few minutes, is one way the nurse can show the patient she cares about him, that she is trying to understand him, and that she respects him.

PATIENT WAYS OF COMMUNICATING AND THE NURSE'S RESPONSES

Patients vary widely in the way they communicate with others. Each patient develops his own pattern of communicating with the nurse. We will discuss some of the different modes of communication patients use. We also will discuss the nurse's responses to these communicative modes.

The Mute Patient

It is difficult for the nurse to know with certainty what a patient who communicates nonverbally is telling her. She has to rely on guess, on intuition, and on her knowledge of and familiarity with the patient in order to figure out his communication. It is important to try to verify her interpretations of the mute patient's behavior. For example, if he stands in front of a locked bathroom door, the nurse might assume that he is telling her he wants to go into the bathroom. She verifies her interpretation by opening the door and watching to see what the patient does. If the patient goes into the bathroom, the nurse can assume that her interpretation is correct. If the patient walks away from the open door, the nurse can assume that she did not interpret his behavior correctly. Thus, one way of finding out if she has understood the mute patient's nonverbal communication is to develop a tentative interpretation, to act on this interpretation if this is possible and not harmful to the patient, and to observe the patient's reaction. With the mute patient there are many situations in which the nurse cannot easily or directly develop an understanding of his communication. For example, if he comes to the nurse and stands in front of her, alternative interpretations can be made of his behavior. Asking him what he wants does not help because he does not answer. However, it might be useful to ask, in order to give the patient an opportunity to reply. If the nurse consistently expects that the patient will not talk, her expectation may encourage him to remain mute. Expecting him to talk by asking him a question without insisting upon an answer, at least will not reinforce his muteness. The nurse might express a guess to the patient as to what she thinks he is telling her. By watching his response she might receive some indication of the correctness of her interpretation. However, it would be inappropriate for the nurse to verbalize guesses on her part, when, for example, she feels uncomfortable in doing so or when they might be disturbing to the patient. We cannot give a formula for the "right" kind of response the nurse should give a mute patient. Her response with the mute patient as with many other patients has to *grow out of the situation* in which she and the patient are participating.

Despite the fact that the nurse may not understand his nonverbal behavior, the patient can have a worthwhile experience with her while they are sitting together in silence or walking together, or while the nurse is helping the patient eat. Emotionally significant and worthwhile experiences that do not involve words are more likely to occur when the nurse has had a continuing relationship with the patient, where she has shown persistent interest, where she accepts the patient, and where the nurse and patient have worked out some mutually satisfactory way of being together.

We have suggested above that nurses often have difficulty *just being with* a mute patient, and we have also suggested some of the reasons. It might be helpful for the nurse to know that the patient's muteness is not willful or deliberate. Rather, it is part of his mental illness—the way he *has to be* at that particular time. There are valid emotional reasons for his not being able to talk. If the nurse can accept this part of his illness—his muteness— without resentment but rather with an inquiring attitude, she might be able to look upon it as a challenge to discover how she can provide opportunities for the patient to begin talking. She can ask herself: How can I participate with him at his own pace, so that he will be able to give up his muteness and find it more satisfying to talk with me? Encouraging the patient to talk may have to be a subtle process. Verbally urging him to do so by coaxing him is likely to have an effect opposite to the one intended. The nurse may have to watch her own responses carefully to find out when to speak to the patient and when to keep quiet; she also may have to watch carefully the patient's responses to her responses. Deep satisfaction awaits the nurse when she can actually help the patient give up his muteness by the situations she creates with and for him.

The Talkative Patient

In contrast to the mute patient is the patient who talks incessantly—who talks a "blue streak." He may say so much so rapidly and in so mixed-up a fashion that the nurse is unable to keep up with or understand him. Even though the patient's talk seems meaningless to the nurse, *it undoubtedly has meaning for the patient*. It is motivated by certain needs, and it is actually saying something. The following questions might help the nurse discover what is being communicated: When does the patient talk in an uninterrupted stream of words, and under what circumstances does he speak differently? The nurse may be able to discover the circumstances that increase the patient's anxiety and lead him to speak excitedly. By removing the anxiety-provoking conditions (if she can) and by allaying his anxiety, she may help the patient talk more intelligibly. What is the pattern of the patient's talk, and does a recognition of the pattern and its variations help the nurse understand the patient? The nurse may learn what is important to the patient by observing his pauses or hesitations at certain words, his emphasis on other words, and his stumbling over others. Without being aware of it, the patient may tell the nurse what words or ideas are important to him. For example, when the nurse asks the patient a question, he may reply with a torrent of words. If the nurse listens carefully, she may be able to pick out a word or a phrase that answers her question. She may do this quite unconsciously, or she may be aware of selecting certain phrases or words. She can try to figure out what in the patient's talk she was able to use to obtain the answer to her question. Was it his tone, the way he looked, or the way he emphasized the important words? In ordinary talk we are always filtering out irrelevant sounds that do not contribute to our understanding. If the nurse can become skilled in such a process of selection, she will be able to distinguish the important words from the unimportant and the meaningful ideas from the meaningless.

When the patient speaks continuously, it is difficult to interrupt and exchange ideas with him. He may have to speak uninterruptedly while the nurse listens to him. But there may be times when she will have an opportunity to inject a brief comment or question. When she does say something to the patient she can notice how he reacts. Does he slow down in his speech? Does he hesitate or stop? Does he hear her statement? What emotional effect, if any, does it have on him? While the patient is talking, if the nurse can keep in mind this question—What is the patient trying to tell me?—she may discover more meaning in his stream of words than she had anticipated.

The Autistic Patient

We suggested in Chapter 5 that the nurse should not leave the impression that she agrees with the autistic patient's delusion. She need not argue with him about his delusion, but might simply make it clear that they do not see eye to eye on this particular issue. However, in rejecting the patient's interpretation of his environment, it is important not to reject the patient. The acceptance of the patient as a person but not of some of his ideas can be conveyed to him by listening carefully to what he has to say and by indicating recognition of his need to talk as he does. It may be that the nurse will have to listen sympathetically to his autistic communication for a long time before he will speak more realistically. The nurse's attitude that the patient's delusional ideas are part of his mental illness and that they can be changed may be very reassuring to him. He may begin to feel that he is "not stuck" with these ideas, and by not agreeing with them the nurse may be able to reinforce whatever disbelief he has about them. In communicating with these patients the nurse is most useful when she is as concrete, down-to-earth, realistic, and specific as she can be on as many topics as possible. Of course, it is unwise for the nurse to maintain the conversation around a patient's delusions when this markedly increases his anxiety or agitation.

It has been our experience that two attitudes toward the patient's communication are not helpful to him: on the one hand, assuming that the patient is impossible to understand and, on the other, believing that you know exactly what the patient means. But we have found it useful to the patient if the nurse assumes that he can be understood, if she considers various possibilities in trying to discover what he means, and if she is willing to ask him what he means and to work with him in order to find out. We have also found that if the nurse can rely on her feelings and can develop a clearer awareness of her feeling responses to the patient, she may learn to "catch on" more easily to the patient's communication.

We have suggested above some of the problems the nurse and patient have in communicating with each other and have examined some of the ways in which the nurse might help make for more effective communication. What are some considerations the nurse might take into account in trying to improve her communication with patients?

The nurse's *tone and manner* are important in responding to the patient. Do they indicate that she appreciates his sensitivities and feelings? Is she trying to fit herself to, and carry on the exchange in, the patient's communicative mode? We have found that a matter-of-fact manner and a tone that indicates interest in and acceptance of the patient often are helpful. *Persisting* with the patient is important; continuing the communicative situation over time holds out the possibility that more stable understandings will develop between them. *Timing of the nurse's response* is also important: Can she gauge when to talk and when to keep quiet, when to take the initiative in the conversation, when to let the patient take the initiative? In the case of a mute patient, the nurse can make the first move and wait for his response. When a communicative exchange has begun with a patient, it is important for the nurse to respond to the patient's response. Her response indicates to the patient that something happens as a result of his efforts, that his actions and words "make a difference" and have some effect on the nurse. It is also important to respond without much delay. Ignoring his response or being uninterested in it may cut off the communication. The nurse might be able to observe what she does to encourage or discourage the patient's response and what the patient does that helps her respond appropriately to him or makes it difficult for her to do so.

The nurse can try to recognize her *anxiety and discomfort* while she is communicating with a patient. For example, does she want to leave the patient as quickly as possible? Does she blame the patient or become angry with him for not communicating with her? With recognition of such feelings she may be able to find ways of reducing her discomfort so that it will not interfere with her communication with the patient. What the nurse says to a patient—the content of her talk—depends on the reason for their communicating with each other at the moment, her relations with the patient, her understanding of him, her comfort with him, and her estimation of what is acceptable to him in the particular situation. *It is unwise for the nurse to lie to a patient.* If he discovers that she has lied to him, it will be difficult for him to trust her in the future. Within the limits set by hospital policy the nurse can try to give the patient as much information as possible. The more information the patient has, the easier it is for him to make a realistic evaluation of his situation. If he becomes aware of or senses concealment and withholding of information, he may become more suspicious or confused. Simple speech, in a form that is comprehensible to him, is essential in communicating with the patient.

Finally, the organization of the ward is an important consideration in achieving effective communication between nurses and patients. Can the ward routine and atmosphere be so arranged that it is possible for the nurse to devote some time to listening to patients? Is she encouraged to do so by her colleagues and do they help her use her imagination in facilitating the patient's communication?

⌐ 14 ⌐

Relating to the Patient

THERE are many facets to the relations the nurse carries on with a patient; these relations involve her actual behavior, her feelings about him and about herself in relation to him, memories about past experiences with him, and expectations about their future behavior with each other. The nurse may have read about the patient's behavior before he was hospitalized and she may have some idea of what he could be like. She might think about ways she can help him and eagerly look for signs that he is different from the way he has been. She may be concerned with whether she is doing the most therapeutic thing for him: Is she getting "too close" to him? Is she sensitive to what he is experiencing? What do restrictions mean to him? In this chapter we shall discuss these and other aspects of the nurse-patient relationship.

GOALS IN RELATING TO PATIENTS

What are the goals the nurse is trying to reach with the patient? She may formulate these goals clearly or she may hold them without being aware of them. Her goals may be specific or very general. In any case, they guide the nurse's behavior with the patient, and she may use them in evaluating her success with him. It is also important for her to be realistic about the possibilities of achieving her goals, for if they are unrealistic she may easily become discouraged and abandon her efforts to help the patient. Once she is clear about her goals and the possibility of achieving them, she can try to discover the best means of reaching them.

The nurse sometimes finds it difficult to accept the fact that she plays an important part in the patient's therapeutic course.

She doubts the significance of her contribution to the patient's welfare and thinks that a change in the patient may have little connection with what she has done; she feels that his improvement or lack of improvement depends exclusively on "what goes on inside him," or is related only to "what the doctor does with him" or to the treatment (shock therapy, insulin therapy, and so forth) that he is receiving. Or she may feel that no matter what she does for some patients, it will not help them because they are hopeless. We believe the contrary: no mental patient with a functional mental illness is hopeless. Further, we hold that the nurse has a central role to play in the improvement of the patient's mental health. We shall try to make explicit the general goals toward which the nurse might work in facilitating the patient's mental health and to identify the more special goals she might try to achieve.

General Goals

In general, the nurse's aim is to *provide opportunities* that will help the patient grow emotionally. She attempts to nourish and to expand the "healthy" part of the patient so that his emotional difficulties are less disabling. This means that she helps the patient gradually to assume more responsibility for himself, to become less dependent, to develop initiative and curiosity, to make his own decisions in a more realistic way, and to make greater use of his capacities and potentialities. She tries to provide the kinds of experiences that will lessen the need for continuing his mentally ill behavior and that will give him a more realistic understanding of himself, his environment, and his relations with others. She takes the patient in as an active participant in their relationship and in the making of decisions about himself. This means that he and the nurse work together toward the achievement of a more productive and satisfying life for him, and toward his greater competence in relating with others.

Specific Goals

The more specific goals the nurse might pursue are complementary to the needs of patients discussed in Chapter 12. That

is to say, for each need of the patient we see a corresponding goal
for the nurse. It is, of course, essential to *maintain the patient
biologically*, to ensure his survival and to protect him against
injury and illness. This means that the nurse tries to protect him
against suicide and against assault by others; that he is provided
sufficient food, clothing, and shelter under proper hygienic conditions; and that he is kept as biologically healthy as possible and
given proper medical care when ill.

A second nursing goal is to *meet the patient's specific and concrete
needs whenever possible*, if meeting such needs will not be injurious
to him and if it will increase his satisfaction or his feelings of
security. This means that the nurse has to discover the particular
object or service the patient wants and provide it in a way that
will be acceptable to him.

Third, the nurse tries to *facilitate the patient's participation with
others*. This means that she relates to the patient as a unique
individual with his own problems that have to be met in a special
way, and that she seeks the type of participation that will be most
useful to him at the moment. In order to do this, she evaluates
the patient's present capabilities. On the one hand, she tries to
avoid activity in which the patient will not participate or is bound
to fail, which would lower his already low self-esteem and increase
his feelings of failure; on the other hand, she does not pursue
activity that is below his capabilities, which would make him feel
he is being treated contemptuously. Determining the appropriate
type of participation is one of the central creative tasks the nurse
engages in with the patient. If the nurse and patient can have a
satisfying exchange, the patient may be able to undertake a
"more mature" type of activity. This means that the nurse must
be ever-ready to respond to the patient's readiness to engage in
a different type of activity. Even when the patient changes very
slowly, the nurse, by being aware of the small changes, may be
able to change her participation with him. If she is able to help
him derive some satisfaction from their relationship, he will have
made an important forward step. In this way he may begin to
reverse a long-standing pattern of avoidance, self-isolation, and
loneliness.

A fourth goal is *facilitating the patient's communication*. It is through communication that he shares the world of others and others share his. Through this mutual sharing, the patient will become more like other people and thereby reduce his mental illness.

Fifth, the nurse tries to *increase the patient's self-esteem*. She relates with him in such a way that he feels more worthwhile, accepted, and respected. Low self-esteem is a major aspect of his mental illness; if his self-esteem is raised, his mental illness will be decreased.

Finally, the nurse tries to *increase the patient's comfort and minimize his anxiety*. Patients suffer much anxiety, which varies from panic to vague discomfort in the presence of others. Sometimes their anxiety is very conspicuous and at other times it is hidden or not easily observable; but it is, nevertheless, present to such a degree that it is an important aspect of their mental illness. The nurse tries to relieve the patient's anxiety when it is particularly severe, and at other times attempts to make the patient as physically and emotionally comfortable as possible. There are times, however, when there is a more important goal than the patient's immediate comfort. For example, it may be more important to disagree with the patient's delusion than to make him momentarily more comfortable by agreeing with it.

We cannot tell the nurse which specific actions will achieve the goals described above. We can only point out the general direction her activities might take. With these guidelines the nurse can try to discover the most appropriate action in her own situation.

In actual practice, it is impossible to achieve one goal without attaining at least some of the others. However, attaining one goal might mean not achieving another; for example, secluding a patient for his protection cuts off his participation with others. The nurse can try to achieve as many as possible of these goals as effectively as she can; if there is a conflict between two or more, she can try to make the choice that is most consistent with the patient's welfare. In any particular situation she may be able to make but a small step toward the attainment of her goals, but it is from cumulative effort to achieve these goals that the patient's mental health will be improved.

IDENTIFYING AND EVALUATING PATIENT IMPROVEMENT

The meaningfulness of the nurse's work and the satisfaction she derives are related to the improvement the nurse sees in the patients in her care. If she sees them "getting better," she feels gratified and encouraged; she is likely to make additional effort to help those who do not appear to be improving; and she is likely to feel that her job is worthwhile. It is, therefore, important for her to be aware of the way she identifies improvement in patients.

From our point of view, a patient has not necessarily improved if he is "better behaved," more "polite," less "noisy," and more "cooperative." However, he may have improved: if he is less anxious—less panicky, agitated, or excited; if he gets along better with other people; if he has fewer symptoms or symptoms that are less severe; if he has more insight into himself; if he communicates with others more easily; if he is better oriented to his environment and is more realistic and effective in dealing with it; if he can carry on relations with others that are more satisfying to him and to them; and if he feels that he is a more worthwhile person. These are, of course, only some of the criteria that may be used in estimating improvement in patients. The nurse may be able to add others.

Though a nurse may be aware of the criteria she uses in evaluating improvement in patients, she may have difficulty in recognizing favorable changes in patients when they do occur. This may be because some patients improve so slowly or because the changes are so minute and subtle that they are easily overlooked. For example, a nurse may fail to notice that a withdrawn patient who ordinarily keeps his head turned toward the wall when others are with him may look quickly and briefly at the nurse when she enters the room. Or the nurse may not see that a patient who has been spoon-fed and urged to accept each bite may, on one occasion, open his mouth without being asked to do so. If the nurse can recognize these slight changes in the patient's behavior, she may be able to develop and expand them into even more significant ones. But if she fails to note the change, she will continue to deal with the patient as if it had not occurred and thus make it more difficult for him to sustain the changed behavior. To the patient, this small change may be a big step and if the nurse fails to notice it, he may become discouraged. Sometimes, a nurse may recognize a major change in the patient but fail to notice an accumulation of small changes. It may be that it is only when the nurse compares the patient's present behavior with his previous behavior that she is struck by the significant change that has occurred.

There are a number of questions that can be raised about what constitutes improvement in patients: How extensive must favorable change be before it is a significant change? How long must it continue before it can be considered a "real" change? If a patient returns to a previous and less effective pattern of behavior, does it mean that he did not "really change"?

We believe that any favorable change in the patient, no matter how small or how temporary, can be considered improvement. We see each forward step of the patient as important even if it is very small or lasts only a few hours or days. It is out of the accumulation of many small and temporary changes that more permanent and more mature ways of behaving will be stabilized. Thus, a patient who has shown increased effectiveness in his relations with others may return to his previous pattern, or he may, as a nurse might say, "slide back." This does not necessarily mean that his constructive experiences are now lost, or that he did not "really improve." It means, rather, that the healthier part of his personality, which was strengthened by satisfying experiences with the nurse, is temporarily dominated by the sicker part of the patient. In this situation, the nurse need not become discouraged. Since she previously was able to reach the patient and to carry on satisfying relations with him, the chances of her doing so again probably have increased. In other words, her previous constructive experiences with him may have left him more accessible and more able to relate to her.

Improvement in patients comes about in *the minute-to-minute relationship nurses or others maintain with a patient* in an immediate situation. Each time a relationship is satisfying and security-giving to a patient, each time he has a constructive experience, it "registers" somewhere in him. *As a result of the continuation and accumulation of these satisfying experiences,* the healthy part of the patient's personality will grow, new personality patterns will emerge, and different ways of thinking and feeling about himself and more mature ways of relating to other people will develop.

The nurse's attitude of hopefulness or discouragement about the possibility of improvement in a patient, or of patients in general, plays a role in identifying improvement and in bringing it about. If she is discouraged and expects no improvement, it will be difficult for her to recognize improvement when it does occur and she will probably not be able to appraise accurately the significance of any change the patient shows. It may be difficult for a nurse to maintain a hopeful attitude toward a patient who has been sick a long time and who has remained relatively unchanged. But it very well may be that the nurse's attitude, and her actions expressing the attitude, that *the patient cannot or will not change,* may contribute to the patient's discouragement and lack of improvement. We have indicated in other parts of this book how the nurse's attitude affects the patient and when it would be necessary for her to change her attitude if she is to facilitate his improvement.

Therefore, it is essential for the nurse to recognize the reasons for her discouragement about improvement in patients. She may become discouraged if the patient takes a long time to show even small changes; if he regresses after having taken some forward steps and suddenly shatters the nurse's new hopes for him; if his improvement is so subtle or slight that it goes unnoticed; or, finally, if she expects rapid changes or frequent signs of her success with a patient and he does not achieve the goals she has set for him.

On the other hand, the nurse's hopefulness that a patient can improve does not ensure improvement. But hopeful attitudes on the part of the staff *create the possibility that the patient's hopeless attitudes about improving will be modified;* when a nurse has a different attitude from that of the patient toward himself, he might begin to change his own attitude. With this change in attitude, some improvement may come about.

Having a generally hopeful attitude about the possibility of improvement in a patient is not the same as having a specific objective the patient must reach within a certain period of time. If the nurse decides in advance just how the patient should change and how quickly this is to be accomplished, she is likely to put pressure on the patient to change in the way she wants and at the pace she desires. Pushing the patient to "get better" may produce resistance and may result in no improvement at all. Here, it would seem that the nurse wants to get a result with the patient because of her own needs. If one is not immediately forthcoming, she may become disappointed or discouraged, may lose interest in him, and may doubt that she "really wants to work with him." If, instead, the nurse believes that the patient can improve and acts on this belief, the healthy part of the patient may grow in their participation with each other.

SENSITIVITY TO THE PATIENT

A nurse's *sensitivity* to a patient is of great value in helping her carry on appropriate activity with him. That is, the "inner" response that she feels with the patient enables her to act in a way that "fits" the particular situation and makes it possible for the relationship to continue with satisfaction for both participants. What makes up this subtle and complex process called sensitivity?

One of the most important aspects of the nurse's sensitivity to the patient, and yet one of the most difficult to define, is *intuition*. At times all nurses depend on their intuition; they may call it a "flash of insight," "a sudden click about the patient's behavior," "a vague hunch about the patient," or "a feeling that something isn't quite right." They mean, in essence, that they have a feeling about what to do or what the patient means without being able to state exactly what it is or without knowing precisely how they came to have this feeling. What has probably occurred is that the nurse has unconsciously registered some communication from the patient, but is aware only of a feeling that she has about him. Although it is difficult to know exactly how this process works, the nurse might learn something about herself, about the patient, and about their relationship if she pays close attention to her intuitive feelings. She might make a conscious effort to recognize them when they occur, to focus on what they are telling her, and to think about how she arrived at the insight that resulted from her feeling. If she can scrutinize her intuitive processes, she might be able to use more effectively the insights gained from them.

Closely related to intuition, and an important element in being sensitive to the patient, is *taking the cue from the patient*. Sometimes a patient gives a nurse only a faint signal or vague indication of what he is feeling or what he wants. If she is willing to wait for such signs and is alert to them when they occur, she may be much clearer about what to do for and with the patient. For example, a nurse may not be sure she is welcome in a patient's room. If she hesitates momentarily at the door, the patient may let her know how he feels about her entering the room. He may "bawl her out" for disturbing him and may block her entrance to the room but, at the same time, he may step slightly to one side of the door. She might accept this movement as an invitation to enter, as a hint that he will accept her presence. In another situation, a nurse might try to start a conversation with a patient who is hallucinating. He may continue his delusional talk without recognizing the presence of the nurse. She might then conclude that he does not want to talk with her. However, if she waits, the patient might suddenly include a few words in his delusional talk that refer to some past activity in which they have engaged. This may be a cue that the patient will talk to her if she gives him enough time; or, perhaps, it might be a hint that he would like to participate with her in the same way he did previously. Taking the cue from the patient involves the following: The nurse is responsive to the patient and is ready to hear his subtle communications. She is willing to let him guide her; she does not necessarily do what he says, but she takes his directions into consideration. She accepts the fact that the patient will tell her in some way what is appropriate in the particular situation.

An important aspect of being sensitive to the patient is *keeping the appropriate distance* from him, both psychologically and physically. For some patients, a warm, friendly approach seems to be indicated. These patients show the nurse that they want some overt demonstration of affection, some "mothering." Other patients need to be approached in a matter-of-fact, down-to-earth manner. For others, considerable reserve is advisable. Paranoid patients are suspicious of friendliness and might become hostile or frightened by too much "closeness." They can accept, and are much more comfortable with, a formal, aloof relationship with the nurse. Open display of warmth might drive the patient away. Similar considerations apply to physical distance or physical contact. Some patients reach out to touch the nurse and very much want to be touched by her. For these patients it is important to make this physical contact; it may reassure them that the nurse is a "real" person. On the other hand, suspicious or frightened patients might interpret physical contact as an attack and be fearful of it. Thus, the nurse must determine when closeness is acceptable and when it is not; she must determine how the patient might interpret and respond to it. In addition to the patient's desires and receptivity, in "getting close to the patient" the nurse must take into account her own feelings of comfort and her own reluctance or hesistancy about physical contact.

Sensitivity to the patient consists of a delicate adjustment and readjustment to him. It develops through familiarity with the patient: knowing him and his ways of acting; knowing which situations arouse his anxiety and which make him feel more comfortable. To be sensitive to the patient means to be "in tune" with him. It means seeing him as a special, unique individual with his own set of sensitivities and patterns of behavior. When a nurse is sensitive to a patient, she is able to put herself in his place, imaginatively and thereby get some idea of what he is experiencing. She is aware of the patient's mood swings and recognizes his ambivalence as shown by his movements toward and away from the nurse: his desire for her companionship and his rejection of it; his wish for affection and his fear of it. If the nurse is sensitive to the patient, she is able to appreciate, on the one hand, his desperate need for help, his intense desire to rely and depend on her, and his wish for a persistent relationship with her; and, on the other hand, his fear and his impulse to be alone in order to avoid the possibility that he might be abandoned by her.

Respect for the Patient

It is generally accepted that respect for the patient is important in the nurse-patient relationship, although it is difficult to state exactly what respect is or how one develops it. What do we mean by respect, and how does one come to respect a patient?

Respect is an attitude toward a patient and a feeling about him that are reflected in the way a nurse approaches and relates to him. It cannot be produced by wanting it or ordering it to appear; it cannot be felt just because "one ought to feel it." Sometimes a nurse earnestly may want to respect a patient, but emotionally she may not feel respectful of him at the time. Feeling inadequate or guilty about her failure to be respectful is not of much use in changing her feelings. It might be more useful for her to try to discover what her attitude is, what stands in the way of her feeling respectful, and how she might overcome these blocks. It might be helpful for her to realize that respect does not come about automatically. Nor does the nurse necessarily start out with a respectful attitude when she first meets a patient. It is likely that the nurse who has many conventional attitudes about mental patients may feel somewhat disrespectful toward patients or that she will have mixed feelings of respect and disrespect. Many nurses begin with a neutral attitude toward patients and come to develop respectful or disrespectful attitudes on the basis of their relations with patients. Respect for a patient may develop when the nurse gets to know him better, shares experiences with him in a personal way, and engages in relations that are satisfying to both of them.

It might be easier to see what respect consists of by considering first what it is not. A nurse is not respectful of a patient when she is revolted by his behavior, is disgusted with him, ridicules him, feels the need to be derogatory toward him, ignores him, is indifferent to him, or is insincere. She is not showing respect for him when she treats him in a stereotyped, artificial, or impersonal way; when she looks upon him as a diagnostic category (a "schizophrenic," for example), as part of the furniture, as part of the mass of patients, or as a piece of protoplasm that is just there.

Respect does not mean that the nurse is conventionally polite to the patient, pities or feels sorry for him, is worried about his welfare or is oversolicitous about his comfort, or that she feels sentimentally attached to him.

When a nurse respects a patient, she *experiences him as another human being not completely different from herself*. Harry Stack Sullivan aptly described this feeling when he said, "We are all more simply human than otherwise." He meant that we are all much more alike than different and that we are all part of the same human situation in which our limitations are greater than our individual accomplishments. In addition to seeing the patient as another human being, the nurse *accepts him as a unique individual* with his own sensitivities, likes, and dislikes, and she relates to him in accordance with this uniqueness. She *sees him as a distinct personality who is worthwhile in himself*—as someone who "counts." She *accepts him for what he is*. She is not moralistic about his behavior and does not establish conditions he must fulfill in order for her to accept him. She can *see his potentialities*. She sees not only what he is now but what he can become. This means that she does not "get stuck" with a picture of the patient that includes only his present state. Rather, she is able to see the healthy part of the patient, which is present in potential; that is, she is able to see aspects of his personality that are undeveloped at the moment but can be helped to grow. The nurse puts her respect into operation when she helps the patient mobilize his drive toward health and when she helps to bring the patient's constructive potentialities into actuality. When she respects the patient, she is able to respond to him on a simple, human level. When she respects him, she derives satisfaction from giving him satisfaction. This does not mean she is overindulgent or self-sacrificing. Rather, she wants to help the patient because she has a genuine interest in him and derives pleasure from contributing to his welfare and doing something worthwhile for him.

Before the nurse can respect the patient, she must respect herself and be respected by her colleagues. If she does not feel worthwhile, she will find it difficult to respect the patient. If other staff members are contemptuous of her, she will find it difficult to respect the patient. Finally, if other personnel are not respectful of the patient, she is likely to adopt their attitudes toward him.

Respect is not an "all-or-none" attitude; nor is it a fixed and unchanging attitude. Rather, respect is a matter of degree and can vary in amount and intensity. The nurse is not ordinarily respectful in the fullest sense of the word all of the time. Sometimes, respect is present to a high degree with some patients and not with others. It may vary with the same patient, depending upon the nurse's mood and the circumstances of the situation. It may vary also with different types of patient behavior. Thus, respect for the patient in the fullest sense is an ideal toward which the nurse can strive.

Treating the Patient as a Child

In relating to a patient who is withdrawn, slow-moving, resistant, indecisive, or who refuses to eat by himself, the nurse sometimes becomes concerned about treating him as a child. For she may have to take the initiative in bathing, in feeding, in making decisions for him about his daily care, or in other ways caring for him as she would a very small child. She may fear that helping him in these ways is disrespectful to him and that her behavior may continue the patient's dependence on her and prevent him from developing emotionally. Or she may be concerned that he will derive so much gratification through her spoon-feeding him, for example, that he will not give up this kind of participation with her. In these situations she finds it difficult to reconcile offering him the opportunity to be dependent upon her with her goal of helping him assume more responsibility for himself.

Part of the problem stems from the difficulty the nurse has in recognizing and accepting the fact that even though the patient is chronologically an adult, there are childish as well as mature aspects to his personality; that is, the patient may be a mixture of child and adult. At times the patient cannot perform effectively in some areas; the childlike aspect predominates and he cannot feed himself. At other times and in other areas, his adult behavior comes to the fore. With this seeming inconsistency in the patient, the nurse has difficulty in accepting his dependent behavior; she feels annoyed that he "behaves like a child" and feels that he "ought to be more adult." Knowing or believing that he can be more adult, she feels guilty or uncomfortable if she spoon-feeds a patient who has consistently been unable to eat by himself. Some of her guilt stems from her training, in which she was taught "not to coddle the patient." Some of her discomfort stems from the fear that "he will never be able to do anything for himself if I do things for him." Her anxiety may be increased by other staff members who tell her she is "making the patient dependent" on her.

In these situations it seems to us that the nurse might profitably direct her attention to finding the behavior that is appropriate to the patient's development and capabilities at the moment, rather than being concerned with whether she is treating him as a child. If she can determine the point at which she can start with the patient, she might be able to participate with the patient in such a way that he gradually gives up his extremely dependent behavior. The question then becomes: Can the nurse relate to the dependent aspects of the patient's behavior in order to bring out more of his adult behavior?

Our experience has been that a nurse may meet the dependent needs of a patient without necessarily making him more dependent upon her. Offering the patient the opportunity to be temporarily dependent upon her is frequently the initial step in helping him assume more responsibility for himself. Meeting the patient's dependent needs is not the same as being oversolicitous, overprotective, or overindulgent with him. Nor does it mean that the nurse should do things for him that he can do for himself. For example, the patient who needs to be spoon-fed may dress himself. If the nurse does things for the patient that he is capable of doing himself, he might feel she is disrespectful of him. Such behavior from the nurse might reinforce the patient's dependence on her. On the other hand, a nurse may try to give a patient more responsibility for himself than he is ready to assume. Her insistence upon treating him as an adult, as an individual who could do things for himself if he wanted to, may "keep him stuck" in a childlike state. Such responsibility may be a burden and may force him to "give up" and become even more helpless.

Thus, the nurse has to discriminate between the actions that will mobilize the patient's initiative and facilitate his growth and those that will not. She can ask herself: "What can the patient do for himself? What are the things he cannot now do alone, and how can I help him so that he will be able to do these things for himself in the future?" The nurse then can carefully observe the consequences of her actions and evaluate them in terms of the kind of patient participation they encourage.

If the nurse can remember that being mentally ill means, in part, that the patient has not handled successfully various phases of the process of maturing and, therefore, has excessively dependent needs (that past deprivations have prevented him from growing up completely), she then can see the process of increasing independence and growth as a gradual one. She can regard the activity she undertakes with the patient as a preliminary step in the expansion of his capabilities. While meeting his dependent needs she can watch for indications that he is ready to take the initiative, make a decision, or take some responsibility for himself. Once he has started some forward movement, the nurse has to be careful not to stand in his way. Her task is to move with the patient at a pace that is acceptable to him and thereby facilitate his taking additional responsibility for himself.

Setting Limits for Patients

In a mental hospital it is inevitable that many limitations will be placed on patient behavior. Patients are kept in the hospital despite their wishes, are prevented from moving about the hospital freely, have to eat and to go to bed at certain times, and so on. In order to function effectively and to protect the patient and society, the hospital sets up a system of rules and routines. Whether the specific rules and routines that exist are the ones that are needed, whether they have to be followed as rigidly as they are in any particular hospital, or whether they are necessarily therapeutic for the patient or exist primarily for the staff's convenience, are all questions that could be explored with profit. Here, we shall discuss circumstances in which the nurse must decide whether to limit the patient's activity and how, when, and where such limitation might be made.

There are numerous situations in which some limitation on the patient's behavior might be required. The patient makes a sexual gesture toward the nurse or tries to kiss or embrace her; he questions the nurse about intimate details of her life; he refuses to bathe for many days in succession; he refuses to get out of bed or wants to eat at a different time or in a different way from the other patients; he exposes himself on the ward or wants to leave the ward dressed inappropriately; he curses at or attacks another patient or a staff member; he does not want to abide by the time limit set for some activity, such as a game, or tries to get the nurse to spend her free time exclusively with him.

In determining whether to set a limit for the patient and what that limit might be, there are a number of considerations the nurse might take into account. The most general is that a nurse cannot be completely permissive or completely restrictive. The realities of the hospital situation and her own feelings do not permit complete permissiveness; and complete restrictiveness would make living unbearable for the patient. Thus, the nurse's attitude about setting limits will be somewhere between these two extremes. Ordinarily, the extent of her permissiveness or restrictiveness will vary from situation to situation, and from patient to patient. For example, she might prevent a patient from attacking another patient but permit him to pace agitatedly up and down the ward. But she might interfere with the agitated pacing of another patient. Such variation in her behavior may be quite appropriate; what may be helpful for one patient may only add to the disturbance of the other.

In deciding on setting limits with a patient, the nurse might take into account his degree of comfort and his feeling of being respected which may result from the limits set on his behavior. For example, if a nurse tells a patient to "keep quiet" when he talks loudly and incoherently to her, she may contribute to his discomfort and feeling of low self-esteem. In another situation, however, setting a limit for a patient might make him feel more comfortable and more respected because the nurse prevents him from humiliating himself. For example, she might stop a patient, even though he objects, from smearing himself with feces.

Sometimes a nurse considers setting a limit on a patient's behavior because she believes that he is trying to "test" or "manipulate" her; she thinks he is trying to see how far he can go before she stops him. Yet, the patient's behavior can be considered in another way. The nurse might feel that the patient cannot help doing what he does. If she interprets the patient's activity as a deliberate maneuver to "get the best of her," her immediate impulse may be to "clamp down on him." If, however, she sees his actions as an aspect of his mental illness and feels that he behaves as he does because of the intensity of his needs, she is likely to set different kinds of limits for him.

In deciding whether to impose a limit on a patient, nurses frequently take into account the consequences. That is, a nurse may know that a patient reacts to a restriction with anger or with a "blowup." To avoid this, the nurse may not restrict the patient or may pass the decision on to someone else. Her fear of the patient or of his blowup may make it difficult for her to consider the realistic requirements of the situation. An awareness of her own reactions may help her in making a more realistic appraisal of the situation and in deciding what will be most beneficial to the patient at that time.

The nurse might also consider her own feelings and attitudes in restricting a patient. She might consider whether setting a limit for the patient is for her own comfort, for her own self-respect, or for her own convenience. When she secludes a patient who follows her around, is she limiting his activities because he annoys her or because she feels he would be more comfortable in seclusion? If she keeps a patient in seclusion for a long time, is it because she does not want to put the effort into helping him stay on the ward, or because other patients are upset by him, or because the patient needs to be alone? We suggest that the nurse's comfort and self-respect is one consideration in setting limits, but there are others that also need to be taken into account.

Sometimes the nurse's comfort becomes the most important factor in deciding on limits for a patient's behavior, with little consideration given to the benefit the patient will derive. On the one hand, if she feels uncomfortable about setting limits, she might be more permissive than is useful for the patient. Such a nurse is anxious about being too strict with a patient. She believes that firmness or restriction will hurt the patient's feelings or will be felt as punishment by him. Therefore, she is reluctant to set limits because "he has suffered so much already." She usually has difficulty saying "No" to the patient and is in great conflict when she has to be firm with him. Because of such attitudes, she sometimes gets into "tight spots" with a patient: she promises or agrees to more than she can produce; she accedes to more than the ward will allow. Sometimes the patient pushes the nurse to further and further extremes without being restricted and becomes very upset in the process.

On the other hand, some nurses find they are most comfortable when they set very strict limits on a patient's behavior, even though these limits may be inappropriate for the patient. They justify this by saying, "The patient must learn to live according to rules and regulations on the outside, so he better learn them here," or "Things will get out of hand if patients do as they wish." These nurses find it difficult to relax the limits they have set, even though doing so might be of distinct benefit to the patient.

Another consideration in setting limits is the effect it might have on the relationship the nurse has with the patient. Sometimes a nurse may feel that prohibition of an activity is a prerequisite for continuing the immediate relationship with the patient. For example, if during a conversation a patient jabs his cigarette repeatedly at the nurse, she will have to take the cigarette away from him if their conversation is to proceed without her being constantly apprehensive, or if she is to remain with him. But if he merely pats her hand, their conversation can continue uninterruptedly. Sometimes a nurse may be reluctant to set limits for the patient because she does not want to "spoil her good relationship with him"; she fears that frustration or restriction by

her will bring about rejection from the patient; or she believes
that the patient "wants" no limits placed on his actions. Often
the patient needs and wants some clear-cut limits that indicate to
him what others will or will not accept from him, what he can or
cannot do with them, and what others will or will not do for him.
Patients often are reassured when a nurse sets a limit for them.
They may feel that the nurse cares about them and is interested
in helping them stop some action of which they later might be
ashamed or which might lower their self-esteem still more. For example, when one patient came into the day room half exposed,
the nurse insisted that she either button her dress fully or go back
to her room. The patient made nò response. The nurse buttoned
her dress and arranged her clothing to cover her adequately.
This was done although the patient protested and resisted the
nurse's efforts. The next day, however, the patient thanked the
nurse for insisting that she be fully dressed.

The nurse has to consider the extent to which she will be able
to maintain the limits she sets for a patient. For example, if the
nurse excludes the patient from an area on the ward that is easily
accessible to him, it may be difficult to enforce the limits she has
set. The nurse might find herself in a continuous struggle with the
patient in an attempt to implement her decision. It is important
for the nurse continuously to evaluate the appropriateness of the
limits she has set. If she discovers that she has made an error in
establishing a limit for a patient, it might be well for her to
abolish the limit and to tell the patient she was in error.

The time at which a limit is set and the nurse's attitude in
setting it are, of course, important. If a particular limit is one of a
series of increasing restrictions, the patient may resist and resent
the limit. If the nurse limits a patient to show him "who is boss,"
he may defy her. He might experience the denial or curtailment
as a "bad authority" depriving him or trying to control him. If
the nurse is harsh, punishing, or retaliatory in setting limits, she is
likely to reinforce his resentment and hatred toward others, increase his negativism, encourage his assaultiveness, or increase his
withdrawal. If she is uncertain in setting limits or in implement-
ing them, she may make it difficult for the patient to accept the

limitation. On the other hand, a limit may be accepted by the patient more easily if the nurse is convinced of its value and expresses her reasons for the limitation, if the nurse-patient relationship has been satisfying, and if the nurse has given the patient as much freedom as possible within the ward context. The nurse might help the patient learn that some limits are inevitable. Through her skill and understanding, she might help the patient learn to deal with authority and to recognize that all authority need not be "bad." She might help him learn that he can accept some limitations without having to withdraw. The patient might come to realize that there is some definite stability in his environment according to which he can regulate his own behavior. This may be of great significance to patients who see their environment as constantly changing and without boundaries or clarity.

In order to increase her understanding of how and when setting limits on a patient might benefit him, the nurse must observe carefully the effect of a particular limit. We present some questions that may be of help in directing her observations: Does the patient feel more comfortable or more respected as a result of the limit, or does it make him more anxious and lower his self-esteem? Does he accept a necessary restriction without becoming more withdrawn and apathetic? Does it help him have a clearer understanding of some of the "rules of behavior"—actions that are acceptable and those that are unacceptable in relating to other people? Does it contribute to greater comfort or stability on the ward of which the patient is a part?

In evaluating the limits that she sets, the nurse needs to keep in mind that the immediate effects are not the only ones to be considered. Often long range effects are difficult to predict, but the nurse might be able to evaluate in retrospect the usefulness of a particular limit. As she continues to observe and to evaluate the effects of the limits set for patients, she will become more skillful in establishing those that are appropriate and for his benefit.

Getting Involved with the Patient

What is meant by "getting involved" with a patient? A nurse might interpret this to mean that she should not get friendly with her patients, should treat them in an impersonal way, and should maintain only minimal contact with them. She might believe that involvement with a patient will be untherapeutic for him and cause difficulties for her. We will examine two kinds of involvement with patients and their possible effects.

The Inevitability of Involvement

In working on a mental hospital ward day after day in close contact with patients who experience strong feelings and show their mental disturbance in overt ways, the nurse is bound to have her feelings "stirred up." Sometimes she will have strong emotional reactions to patients. At other times her feelings may be less intense. She may experience compassion, pity, tenderness, affection, or concern; she may feel anger, fear, anxiety, or disgust. These emotional reactions seem to be unavoidable. Being human, the nurse will respond to the strong emotions patients show. She may not want to have such feelings and may deny that she has any emotional reaction to patients. Sometimes she may realize she has such feelings but may try not to show them or may attempt to push them out of her mind. Or, without being aware of it, she may try to hide her feelings and may even succeed in convincing herself that she is detached and untouched emotionally. However, if she observes herself closely, she may recognize that the strong feelings of patients do affect her. This effect is not always readily evident: when a patient is disturbed, the nurse may react only by blanching or becoming flushed. At times she may reveal the impact of the patient's feelings on her in a dramatic or direct way. She may burst into tears or become very upset; she may suddenly show considerable anger at what appears to be a minor incident; she may become involved in a heated argument with other staff members about a patient.

Thus, it would seem that rather than trying to convince herself and others that she has no "feelings about" or "involvement with" a patient, the nurse might attempt to discover what her feelings are, how intense they are, and what she ordinarily does with and about them. That is, she might try to discover how she shows or conceals her feelings and how she acts when they are present. Once she recognizes that she has feelings about patients and becomes aware of the nature of her emotional involvement, then she can ask herself how it can be handled therapeutically for the patient. We are suggesting that *it is inevitable that the nurse will become involved with patients in the sense of being emotionally affected by them.*

Kinds of Involvement

In discussing the nature of the nurse's involvement with patients, it might be useful to distinguish between two types of involvement. The first can be called *distorted involvement,* in which *the nurse uses the patient primarily for her own emotional needs and purposes.* The second type can be called *sympathetic involvement.* Here, *the nurse shows interest in the patient "for the patient's sake" and welfare and because she wants to have a satisfying relationship with him.*

Below is an illustration of an extreme case of *distorted involvement.*

Miss Albans developed a close relationship with Mr. Bell while she was a nurse on the ward. During the course of their relationship she said she had "peculiar feelings about him" and thought she was "in love with him." At the same time she felt very "mixed up" about him, since she realized he was sick. Her feelings affected her behavior toward him and toward other patients. When he was upset, she would get upset. If another patient agitated him, she became very angry at the other patient. When she tried to give him special attention, he tried to make love to her. Only with great effort could she turn this down. She believed that he sensed her feelings and that he used various devices to break down her resistance. When she told him she was a nurse, had to attend to his needs, and could not make love to him, he would insist that she did not like her job anyway. He would appeal to her sympathy by saying that nobody ever paid any attention to him and that he was very much mistreated and very unhappy.

When Mr. Bell's transfer to another ward was being discussed, Miss Albans favored the transfer and intended to speak for it at a meeting of nursing personnel. However, during the meeting she found to her amazement that she was supporting his staying on the ward. She recognized that she was doing this for her own needs, in order to have him near her. She then seriously began to doubt her ability to help him.

Miss Albans could not speak freely about her problem nor could she resolve it. She became more and more confused and unable to handle her feelings. The situation became so difficult for her that she finally resigned.

In the case described above, the nurse used the patient for her own emotional needs and ends. The nurse became aware of this fact, but only after she had experienced much difficulty with her feelings. Often a nurse may be quite unaware or only partially aware of what she is doing with a patient. Sometimes, she may deliberately use the patient to "work out" or "act out" her personal problems. In either case she has a distorted view of what she can expect from the patient and what she can give to him. She may have difficulty setting limits for the patient or saying "No" to him, even though she believes that he would benefit if she did so.

There are other indications of a nurse's distorted involvement with a patient. Among them are the following: The nurse is excessively worried about him; she feels intense hatred for him; she is preoccupied with him to the exclusion of other patients or constantly is "overcome with pity" for him; she is so possessively attached to a patient that she resents anyone else's relationship with or interest in him; she feels that no one else can nurse him as well as she can; she frequently is upset when he is upset or when "things don't go right" for him. She may think that others are jealous of her relationship with the patient and that they want to "break it up." She may find it difficult to accept anyone else's point of view concerning her activities with the patient.

In this type of involvement the nurse's feelings make it difficult for her to distinguish between activities that will be of value to the patient and those that will not be. As a result, her feelings prevent her from being of benefit to the patient.

The illustration in Chapter 11 is an example of *sympathetic involvement*. As the aide developed her relationship with the patient, she responded to him with warmer and friendlier feelings, with greater spontaneous interest and tenderness, with more genuine concern for his welfare. In general, in this type of involvement, the nurse is able to sympathize with the patient and yet not "lose herself" in him or in his problem. She can be objective about their relationship without being impersonal. She does not use her role as a nurse to keep her distance from the patient or to hide her feelings about him from herself. She can see the realistic limits of their relationship and can maintain warmth and sympathy within these limits. She can carry on a relationship "that matters" to both. Her involvement facilitates a continuing relationship with the patient in which his satisfaction, security, and self-esteem are increased. The nurse does not regard the patient as "exclusively hers," but is gratified if her relationship with him enables him to form more satisfying relations with others. Finally, she derives satisfaction from seeing the patient increase in his self-esteem and develop greater satisfaction in living.

In trying to develop sympathetic involvement with a patient, a nurse may have a number of difficulties. First, she may have a problem with herself. She may feel anxious about "getting too close" to the patient; she may fear she might become upset or might become too much like the patient if she gets to know him too well. Thus, some of her own emotional difficulties may make it necessary for her to keep "distance" between her and the patient.

Second, the patient may present some difficulties. As the nurse "gets closer" to him, he may become more disturbed. Because he has lived in isolation and loneliness for so long, he may be unable to accept the nurse's warmth and interest without some disbelief, fear, or upset.

Third, the nurse may have problems with other staff members. They may feel she is showing favoritism to a particular patient or that she is "making him dependent" on her. They may envy her relationship with the patient or resent her because she has the kind of relationship with him that they feel they cannot develop. They may feel threatened because by comparison they appear to be inadequate.

Finally, the institution may make it difficult for her to develop a sympathetic and close relationship with the patient. Persons in authority in the hospital may frown upon the nurse's spending so much time with a patient. The hospital routines and regulations and her other duties may leave her little time to form such a relationship.

If a nurse is to develop a meaningful relationship with a patient, she can do so only by having an emotional interest in him and by developing sympathetic involvement with him. If she tries to be detached or impersonal in her relations, she may reinforce his isolation and withdrawal. Many patients are accustomed to keeping their distance from other people by indifference, by active hostility, or by hiding or not acting on their friendly feelings. If the nurse remains aloof from a patient, she may make it difficult for him to come out of his "shell" and share meaningful experiences with her. If she keeps her distance from him, she will not afford him the opportunity to develop relations with another that may be satisfying and of benefit to him.

CONVENTIONAL ATTITUDES AND EXPECTATIONS

Certain attitudes and expectations that are common in our relations with persons outside the hospital may be inappropriate in relating with patients. Sometimes it is difficult for the nurse to recognize that these attitudes and expectations enter into her relations with patients and that they stand in the way of her functioning effectively.

One conventional attitude that may be especially troublesome is the nurse's tendency to evaluate patient behavior in accordance with moral standards of right and wrong and good and bad. Thus, a nurse might consider an assaultive patient bad and feel that he should be punished. She might think a patient who exposes his genitals is immoral. She might consider him disgusting when he spits at her or when he urinates on the floor. Ordinarily, such behavior is disapproved of, rejected, or condemned outside the hospital because it violates our moral code, and the nurse carries these attitudes into the hospital. She learned these moralistic attitudes at an early age and has been using them for a long time; they are very much a part of her thinking and feeling about people. Therefore, they arise almost automatically in her relations with patients. She takes these attitudes so much for granted that she may not be fully aware of them and realize that they affect her relations with patients. These attitudes seem so natural and inevitable that she has difficulty imagining a different reaction to the patient's behavior.

There are other attitudes that fit into and accompany these moralistic attitudes. Usually the nurse also feels that the patient is capable of controlling his unconventional behavior; she thinks he is deliberately engaging in unconventional behavior in order to be "mean and nasty." The fact is that *the patient cannot help or control* many of the things he does. If the nurse could look upon the patient as *a sick person who has to do* many of the things he does and *who is doing what he is able to at the moment*, she might not continue to feel so critical or condemnatory of him. Just as a patient with a broken leg cannot run or an exhausted patient cannot rise from his bed, the mentally ill person cannot help his unconventional behavior. If the nurse accepts the idea that the patient cannot control many of his activities, she can then seek an alternative to reacting to him moralistically.

One such alternative is for the nurse to react to his unconventional behavior in a matter-of-fact way, to become curious about it, and to try to understand it. In contrast to feeling that the patient's behavior is wrong or disgusting or that it should be prohibited or punished, she can try to understand how and why it occurred. *She can try to figure out what it means to the patient, how she and other staff members respond to it, what effect these responses have on the patient, and what can be done to change the patient's behavior so that it is more satisfying to him and to personnel.*

It is important for a number of reasons to find an alternative to the moralistic attitude in relating with patients. The patient may have been criticized, condemned, and rejected in the past, and these attitudes may have contributed to his illness. A blaming and punishing attitude may reinforce his loneliness and hopelessness by confirming his feeling that people cannot or will not understand him. These moralistic attitudes might take the nurse's attention away from the patient's needs and from her relations with him and direct it toward her own feelings. She may become so "tied up" by her condemnatory feelings that she cannot find ways of establishing satisfying relations with the patient.

Another reaction that may be troublesome to the nurse is her tendency to react personally to the patient's behavior. If he curses, physically attacks, or derogates or mocks her, she feels rebuffed, insulted, and hurt. It is not unusual to want to retaliate when one has been insulted, but the patient may be attacking the nurse because *he has to attack someone*, and she just happens to be there. His anger or hatred toward her may be quite irrational and related not to her but to past injustices he has suffered. The patient attacks the nurse not because of who she is but because, in his mind, she stands for someone else. In this sense he is not attacking the nurse personally, and if she could see his behavior as part of his mental illness she might not have to react to it as if it were a personal affront.

Not only does the nurse have conventional attitudes and expectations of the patient, but she also has them of herself. She may be concerned about doing the "right" thing with the patient and try to act as she thinks the authorities in the hospital want her to act. She may fear disapproval, blame, or punishment if she acts differently. She may want to follow a prescribed course of action with a patient in order to avoid mistakes and criticism. She may hope that she will be given specific directions on how to relate with a patient in order to achieve a desirable result. Implicit in these attitudes is the expectation that there is "one way" or a "right" way to approach the patient and that the person in charge can tell her what it is. This implies that there is a mechanical, direct, and easily specified way to relate with patients and that all the nurse need do is follow the directions given her.

The fact of the matter is that there is no preestablished course the nurse can follow to ensure success with a patient. If she becomes preoccupied with what she "ought to" be doing, with how others are judging her actions, or with whether she is doing the "right thing," it will be difficult for her to focus on her relations with the patient. The nurse often may have to search gropingly for the appropriate action. From our point of view, *a nurse's relations with a patient are evolving ones.* In the course of relating with the patient, she builds on her previous experiences with him and discovers new ways of participation. If the nurse is to develop more useful ways of relating with the patient, it is important that her attitudes and expectations of *what she should be able to do with and for the patient do not stand in the way of what she can do with him.*

SELECTIVE ATTENTION

In relating with patients it is inevitable that the nurse will pay attention to some parts of a patient's behavior and personality and ignore others. That is, without knowing it, she will concentrate on certain aspects of the patient and overlook others. She will look for certain things in the patient and avoid looking for others. Where she focuses her attention and places her emphasis plays an important role in her view of the patient and influences the actions she undertakes with him. Therefore, it might be useful for the nurse to become aware of how she *selectively attends* to the patient.

There are two major ways in which a nurse might think about a patient. She might think in terms of his "sick" or his negative behavior, and she might focus on his "healthy" or positive ways of acting. By "sick" or negative behavior we mean his unconventional, hostile, contemptuous, displeasing, autistic, or destructive behavior. By "healthy" or positive behavior we mean the tender, kindly, respectful, rational, cooperative, and constructive activity he undertakes. Though patients in mental hospitals engage in much negative behavior, they do not do so all the time. Because the negative aspects are so much a part of the patient's way of living, often the nurse pays attention only to these aspects, sees the patient almost exclusively in these terms, and acts as if he engaged only in negative behavior. By doing this she overlooks or ignores aspects of the patient that may be different from the picture she has of him.

In Chapter 1 we discussed selective attention in the nurse's attitude toward the "assaultive patient" and pointed out that the nurse tended to remember only the assaultive incidents and disregarded the times the patient was not assaultive. In emphasizing and magnifying his assaultiveness, she "blocked out" the rest of his behavior. Thus, she did not see the patient "as a whole."

A similar process might occur with an autistic patient. If she thinks of him as delusional and has experienced a considerable amount of autistic talk with him, the nurse might find it difficult to focus on his more rational behavior. This might be especially true if the rational behavior occurs less frequently than the autistic behavior.

It is easy for the nurse to focus on negative aspects of a patient's behavior and to overlook positive aspects. The negative behavior is conspicuous and in some form is very often present. This behavior arouses intense emotional reactions in the nurse, is troublesome, and must be dealt with by her. Because a patient's negative behavior becomes so important to nurses, they emphasize it in their discussions with each other; and this tends to keep their attention focused on it. For example, if at change of shifts a nurse describes in detail the attacks, upsets, or disagreeable behavior in which patients have engaged even though the ward was quiet and pleasant part of the day, attention is not only focused on the negative but the nurse hearing the report may develop an expectation that she will have to deal with negative behavior on her shift. She might look for such behavior or even unknowingly help to bring it about. On the other hand, patients' positive behavior often is not reported fully at change of shifts but tends to be dismissed with the phrase: "Everything was all right."

As a consequence of focusing her attention on the negative aspects of patients' behavior, the nurse may develop a distorted picture of a patient; she does not see him in perspective or may see him as much sicker than he really is. She may become discouraged about the patient and feel that it is impossible for him to change. Because she sees only his sick behavior, she may not give him responsibilities that he might be able to handle. Not experiencing his positive, healthy side, she does not try to figure out ways of helping it grow. Thus, she may not offer him opportunities to relate in other than a sick way and may not encourage him when he demonstrates healthy behavior.

If the nurse can become aware of the ways in which she focuses her attention on the negative aspects of the patient, she may be able to develop a more realistic, balanced appraisal of his assets and liabilities. When she is not preoccupied with the negative to the exclusion of the positive, she may be able to see the patient more as he actually is and as he can become. Once she recognizes and pays attention to the healthy, positive aspects of the patient, she can seek them out in order to facilitate their growth.

STEREOTYPED RESPONSES TO PATIENTS

When a nurse begins to work on a mental hospital ward, in addition to having many other feelings, she may be surprised, curious, or puzzled about a patient's behavior. It has a kind of newness and interest for the nurse which is a challenge to her. She may regard it as a problem that she could solve if she understood the patient better. As time goes on the patient's behavior may lose its newness or problematic quality. The nurse becomes accustomed to it and in some way "adjusts" to it. This adjustment may take the form of *stereotyped responses*. That is, the nurse develops a few routinized, automatic approaches to the patient and repeatedly deals with him in the same way. A nurse's stereotyped responses to a patient are of little value to him. We will try to understand what these responses are, how they arise, and what effects they might have.

There are many kinds of stereotyped responses to patients. For example: The patient repeats words and phrases and the nurse consistently responds by not listening. The patient speaks in a vague, elusive way, and the nurse automatically dismisses his talk as nonsense or "crazy." The patient twirls his finger in the air interminably, and the nurse repeatedly feels annoyed and expresses her annoyance with the phrase, "Oh, *that* again." The patient regularly is incontinent, and the nurse labels him "a soiler" and expects his incontinence to continue. The patient's talk is difficult to understand, and she mechanically refers to him as "paranoid."

These stereotyped responses can develop around any activity with patients. An illustration is given below of such a response around tube-feeding.

A patient was tube-fed over a period of months, and the nurse repeatedly approached him with the expectation that "he won't eat." This expectation became automatic and routine, as were the preparations she made for tube-feeding him. The patient always was efficiently packed, and the tube-feeding tray was expertly prepared. The nurse never offered the patient food or asked him if he would like to drink the preparation. She mechanically gave the tube to the doctor, and the patient was regularly fed by him.

In the situation described above, the nurse expected the patient to be the same each day as he was the day before, never anticipating any change. Her stereotyped attitude became evident both in her notes and in her verbal descriptions of her activity with him. The nursing notes read: "Patient was tube-fed. Cooperative. Tube-feeding retained." With this stereotyped approach the nurse saw no possibility of change and presented no opportunity for change to occur. She failed to observe what was going on with the patient at the moment; she did not look for cues that he might have been ready to eat another way; she did not talk with or about him to learn if he could behave differently, or try to encourage him to eat without the tube-feeding; she did not explore in her imagination alternative ways in which she might influence him to change his behavior.

Stereotyped responses are also indicated by the way a nurse talks to a patient. When a patient asks the nurse why he should do something which she asks of him, the nurse may reply: "It's good for you." "The doctor ordered it." "It will get you well." "Because I want you to." "Because I tell you to do it." None of these responses is necessarily stereotyped, but if her answer is given in a mechanical way as a substitute for a more reasonable and considered explanation, the response may easily become stereotyped. Behind the nurse's automatic responses to a patient may be equally stereotyped attitudes. She may feel: "He's just crazy." "He's a manipulator." "He's a troublemaker." "He could do better if he wanted to." When a nurse labels a patient and thinks of him primarily in terms of that label, when she continually uses clichés in describing him, or when she responds to him in a restricted way, she does not see him as a whole person, with potentialities for many different ways of behaving. Nor is she using her imagination to find different, less obvious aspects of the patient's personality.

What are the reasons for the development and maintenance of stereotyped responses? Sometimes the patient himself contributes to the nurse's developing stereotyped responses to him, as illustrated in the following situation.

A patient repeatedly mimicked the actions and words of nurses, almost duplicating them. He also followed nurses around the ward, copying their gestures. If they turned to look at him, he grinned and leered in an embarrassed way. Most of the nursing personnel responded in the same way to this behavior. They became uncomfortable, automatically grinned back at him, and attempted to get away as quickly as possible. This unvarying response continued for many weeks until it was pointed out to nursing personnel by someone who was not a regular member of the ward staff. Even after they became aware of their stereotyped response, personnel had difficulty changing their behavior.

In the situation described above, the patient's stereotyped behavior was so rigid and compelling that it virtually "forced" nursing personnel to respond in a reciprocally stereotyped way. Thus, a stereotyped process was established in which each helped to continue the stereotyped response of the other.

Frequently, a stereotyped response develops and continues because it is the easiest way for the nurse to handle a patient. If she can follow a cut-and-dried procedure, there is something definite for her to do. Such a routine gives her a feeling of security, for it is less anxiety-provoking to follow a routine than to try out new ways of dealing with a patient or to try to imagine how to do something different with him. The stereotyped way becomes the comfortable and the familiar way.

Sometimes, the nurse takes over, or is taught, a stereotyped response to the patient by other personnel. It may be traditional to deal with a patient or with all patients in a particular way; or certain ways of handling patients may be accepted and approved. In such cases, the nurse does what is expected because she wants the approval of her colleagues. She continues to approach patients in the accepted way because others have done it that way in the past or because she assumes that since patients have been handled in a certain way for so long a time "it must be the right way." Stereotyped responses take on the appearance of being "the only way to do things" and "the natural and easy way to deal with the patient." Yet, there are different "natural" ways of doing things in different hospitals.

Another way the nurse develops a stereotyped response is to "fall into" or "pick up" this mode of behavior and continue it without quite knowing how she is behaving or why she acts in this manner. Ordinarily, the nurse does not question the value of her stereotyped reactions, and this makes it easy for her to continue to use them.

What are the effects of stereotyped responses? These responses tend to make nursing relatively ineffective and even dull and uninspired. Routine and automatic ways of thinking, feeling, and participating with patients may become so standardized and rigid that the nurse cannot get a fresh view of them or deal with them in a different or original way. Her preconceptions and ready-made responses limit her imagination, and she is unable to see alternative ways of acting. Her responses lack spontaneity and may not be appropriate to the situation. In addition to maintaining the nurse's job as dull, boring, and uninspired, stereotyped responses also may have untherapeutic effects for patients. Part of the patients' mental illness consists of their stereotyped patterns of relating to others. Such patterns bring patients little satisfaction and are difficult to alter. When the nurse cannot see new ways of relating to them, she cannot help them change their "sick" ways of behaving. When she approaches them in a *stereotyped way, with the image that they will continue to be the same*, she contributes to keeping them as they are. If she treats them as if they will be unchanged and cannot change, they will not change. Thus, she helps to stabilize these aspects of their mental illness and also reinforces their feelings of hopelessness about changing. In such a static situation, it becomes difficult for the nurse to profit from her experiences with patients, and they do not profit from their relations with her.

We are not suggesting that the nurse attempt to abolish all routines. Routines are necessary for the effective organization of a ward and play a part in providing patients good nursing care. But good organization is not the same as stereotyped and routine responses to patients. To emphasize a statement already made, it is important that the nurse does not develop a stereotyped attitude and approach to all patients, dealing with them in a mechanical and automatic way, and viewing them as part of a mass. An effective organization might provide the nurse the time and inclination to respond to individual patients in a personal, spontaneous way.

If the nurse is to change her stereotyped approach, she must become aware of it, develop some dissatisfaction with it, and try to understand the reasons for continuing her stereotyped responses. She then might be able to look at the patient not only in terms of what "he now is" but also of what "he was" and of what "he can be." If she can overcome the compelling effect the patient has upon her as he relates to her at the moment, which makes it difficult for her to see him as he was and as he can be, she might not have to "get stuck" with her stereotyped conception of and response to the patient. Thus, she may not have to contribute to keeping him the way he is and may be able to help him change.

ANXIETY IN RELATING TO PATIENTS

It is inevitable that the nurse frequently will experience anxiety in her relations with patients. Her anxiety will vary in intensity. It may continue for only a short time or it may persist for a relatively prolonged period. She may be only dimly aware of it or she may feel it acutely. Whatever its form at any particular time, she must handle it in such a way as to prevent it from seriously impairing her effectiveness with patients. Some consideration of the possible sources of anxiety and the nurse's response to it might help her handle it.

The general condition of the ward might be a source of anxiety for the nurse. When the level of tension is high and the ward disturbed, her anxiety may be stimulated. Sometimes this is expressed by a statement such as: "When I come into that tense atmosphere, I get jumpy myself."

The kinds of situations in which the nurse and patient participate that produce anxiety in the nurse were described in Part I. We indicated that the nurse might become anxious when she is trying to deal with a patient who is in panic, is extremely anxious, is hostile or assaultive, is mute or withdrawn, and so on. In each of these situations, although it may be contrary to the wishes or intentions of the patient, his feelings and behavior might evoke anxiety in the nurse. Previous difficult experiences with a patient may contribute to the nurse's anticipation of anxiety. Sometimes this anticipation of anxiety may contribute to bringing it about. A striking characteristic of anxiety is the circular fashion in which it can operate and the ease with which both patient and nurse can reinforce anxiety in each other. The nurse's apprehension is conveyed to the patient, who becomes anxious in response to her anxiety; and the patient's anxious response stimulates further anxiety in the nurse.

The nurse's relations with her colleagues may be another source of anxiety for her. Misunderstandings, disagreements, and conflicts between ward personnel may provoke anxiety in the nurse. She may not get the emotional support she wants or needs from her colleagues; or she may not get the kind of instruction she wants from persons in authority. When her colleagues "let her down," she may become more readily susceptible to anxiety.

When the nurse is extremely anxious with a patient, a common response is to withdraw from him or to try to escape from the situation. If she does not avoid the patient, she may find that she has difficulty in focusing on him because she is preoccupied with herself. Or her view of the patient may become distorted or unclear, and she may become unable to judge what he wants or needs, or what seems to be going on with him. She may find that her relations with him are inappropriate, that she is hesitant and uncertain with him, that her imagination is blocked, and that, generally, she is ineffective with him.

If a nurse repeatedly experiences anxiety with a patient, it may be difficult to maintain a sympathetic attitude toward him. She may easily become angry, want to punish him, show a great deal of impatience, and become more arbitrary in her relations with him. She may become impervious to his suffering or only fleetingly aware of it. She may become indifferent to it and minimize or dismiss it. When she responds in these ways, she is trying to protect herself against the discomfort of the anxiety.

If the nurse is to develop some effectiveness in handling her anxiety and minimizing its interference in her relations with patients, she must be able to identify it in herself when it arises. This means that when she is anxious, she admits it to herself instead of denying it or feeling that it will go away if she ignores it. Once she recognizes her anxiety, she can try to discover its source, and the kinds of situations that increase it. She also might direct her attention to her characteristic ways of dealing with anxiety, especially when it arises in her relations with patients. Does she withdraw into the nursing station? Does she busy herself with an activity, such as making the ward look spotless? Does she begin to blame or attack others for not doing their jobs? Does she become restrictive with the patient? Does she become discouraged and hopeless about patients? Does she feel concerned about her adequacy as a nurse?

When the nurse's anxiety arises in her relations with patients, *she might use it as a cue* that something important is happening between her and the patient which she might observe more closely. She might try to discover the point at which her anxiety increased and ask herself how and why her anxiety mounted at this time. She might try to recall similar situations in which her anxiety was aroused, compare them, and try to discover what they have in common. It may help her to deal with her anxiety if she asks herself questions about it, instead of protesting that "it shouldn't be" or denying that it exists.

When the nurse is anxious, it is especially important for her to feel supported and respected by her colleagues. They can help her manage her anxiety in her relations with patients by providing an opportunity for her to unburden herself and to discuss the details of a situation that provoked her anxiety. Lending a sympathetic ear and being accepting and supportive of her when she is anxious helps to relieve and reduce her anxiety.

SUMMARY

In Part II we have attempted to increase the nurse's awareness and understanding of her interpersonal relations with patients. We have discussed different aspects of the nurse-patient relationship and the factors that influence it. We hope that an increased awareness and understanding of these processes will help the nurse develop greater freedom to explore alternative ways of dealing with patients, to use her imagination in discovering new ways of meeting patients' needs appropriately, and to increase her facility in contributing to the improvement of patients' mental health.

We have attempted to show how patient and nurse affect each other. In the nurse-patient relationship the nurse might grow in her understanding of the patient and of herself and find experiences with patients satisfying and maturing. Or she might grow very little in the course of her work and look upon her job as routine, difficult, and promising little satisfaction. Similarly, the patient might slowly establish trust and faith and gradually improve his mental health. Or his mentally ill behavior might continue and be reinforced. The benefit derived by both depends on the kind of interpersonal relations they carry on with each other.

We wish to point out that the interpersonal processes we have described—understanding, communicating, and relating to patients—go on simultaneously, yet each grows out of the other, with an earlier aspect of one process affecting a later aspect of another. In an actual situation, these processes are difficult to separate. We have discussed them separately only in order to examine them in detail. We have not, of course, discussed everything relating to these processes; the nurse may be able to point out many things that we have omitted or have not emphasized sufficiently.

In trying to determine whether and how our analysis and approach is applicable in her own hospital, the nurse might remember that she does not necessarily have to create a special situation to maintain relations with the patient. She can communicate with a patient while she is serving his meal; she can try to understand him while she is giving him medication; she can carry on a relationship with him while they are making beds together. The nurse also might remember that if she has only a few minutes to spend relating to a patient, instead of the long periods of time she might like to have available, even these few minutes can be of benefit to him.

In reading our description of some of these interpersonal processes, such as sensitivity to the patient and respect for him, some nurses may feel that it is too difficult or even impossible to achieve the type of understanding and to develop the ways of dealing with patients that we have suggested. Therefore, they may feel inadequate or discouraged. Such a reaction might be avoided if the nurse regards our discussion as an attempt to stimulate thinking about the part she can play and the standards toward which she might strive in trying to maximize the therapeutic usefulness of her interpersonal relations with patients.

« 15 »

Conclusion

THERE is no easy method for dealing effectively with patients, nor is there one type of nurse-patient relationship that
invariably will contribute to the patient's improvement. Nursing
the mentally ill is a complex, difficult, and demanding task if it is
to result in therapeutic benefit for the patient. Therefore, it is
important that the nurse develop a way of thinking about her
nursing situation and a way of looking at the nurse-patient relationship. Throughout the book we have tried to supply a frame
of reference that might help the nurse organize her experiences
with patients. It might be useful to summarize briefly our approach to the nursing of patients in the mental hospital.

If the nurse is to increase her contribution to patient improvement, we believe she has to become an *acute observer*, who maintains an active curiosity and a habit of asking questions about her
own and the patient's feelings and behavior and an interest in
developing insight into her own and other persons' stereotyped
ways of thinking about and behaving with patients. The careful
observation of small changes in a patient that could be built upon
and expanded is a significant part of this process. The nurse's
observation of the patient might include an attempt to see him in
a number of different ways and from a variety of viewpoints. Her
observations of herself might include an examination of her attitudes, feelings, and reactions to the patient, to authority figures
in the hospital, and to her colleagues. She might also observe the
situations in which she and the patient find themselves and the
ways in which their mutual participation makes these situations
what they are. The nurse can examine what she does with the
patient, what he does with her, and the cumulative effect on the

patient of their interaction with each other. Finally, the nurse might look at the social context—the rules, policies, procedures, and customary patterns—to see how the components of the social context operate.

Once the relevant observations have been made, the nurse can try to *evaluate and appraise* the therapeutic effects of the factors she has been observing. During this appraisal the nurse can try to determine which aspects of the situation seem to maintain the patient's mental illness and which seem to facilitate his mental health. She might then explore *alternative ways* of changing those aspects she feels need to be altered. In exploring various alternatives, she can *permit her imagination to roam freely over various possibilities*, no matter how unrealistic, unusual, or impossible they appear to be. After she has let her imagination wander, she can narrow the alternatives to those that are realistically possible and decide what kinds of changes in her relations with patients she would like to undertake.

Once a change has been decided upon, the nurse can try to determine the appropriate way of instituting the change. She can try to strike a balance between a definite and specific plan for dealing with the patient and leaving the way open for spontaneous participation with him and for permitting herself to change the plan if this seems necessary. When the nurse has actually instituted a change or a series of changes over a period of time, she can then *evaluate the effects of her intervention*. On the basis of this appraisal she might decide to continue with the patient along lines already begun or to proceed in another direction.

The approach we have been suggesting is a continuous process of asking questions, obtaining tentative answers, making the indicated changes, asking more questions, evaluating the changes, and making further changes when necessary. It involves curiosity, persistence, and patience in seeking therapeutic ways of participating with patients. We are suggesting that the nurse become a participant observer who is able to see the patient as he is and as he might become, and is able to evaluate the nurse-patient relationship as it presently is constituted and as it might develop in the future. We also suggest that the nurse discuss the details of her observations, evaluations, and interventions with her colleagues. Increased insight and imaginative ways of participating with the patient might grow out of these collaborative efforts with her colleagues and the nurse might learn to deal with the patient more appropriately and thereby contribute to his satisfaction, his security, and his improved mental health.

INDEX

Index